METROPOLITAN MEDICAL CENTER

Medical Terminology and
Machine Transcription Course

2nd Edition
Frederick J. Frensilli, M.D., F.A.C.S.

Clinical Professor of Urology
George Washington University School of Medicine
Washington, DC

CONTRIBUTING EDITOR

Carolee G. Sormunen
University of Northern Michigan

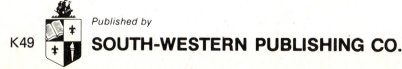

K49

Published by
SOUTH-WESTERN PUBLISHING CO.

CINCINNATI   WEST CHICAGO, IL   DALLAS   PELHAM MANOR, NY   PALO ALTO, CA

Copyright © 1985
by South-Western Publishing Co.
Cincinnati, Ohio

The text of this publication, or any part thereof, may not be reproduced or transmitted in any form or by any means, electronic or mechanical, including photocopying, recording, storage in an information retrieval system, or otherwise, without the prior written permission of the publisher.

ISBN: 0-538-11490-8
Library of Congress Catalog Card Number: 83-51012

456H21098
Printed in the United States

PREFACE

This course is an exciting introduction to the world of medicine through the machine transcription of medical case histories. It is not designed to teach you everything about medicine and medical words, but it will begin your study of the fascinating terminology used in this critical, high-tech, and stimulating world. You will study individual medical terms along with their definitions. You will be hearing them and typing them in context. This way you will readily develop a base for understanding and using all medical words and phrases. With additional study and practice this understanding and use will continue to grow.

When you first start, the sounds and words of medical practice will be strange to you. As you study them and their roots or origins, your confidence will build. Gradually, medical jargon, which has always seemed mysterious, will become understandable and fascinating.

F.J.F.

CONTENTS

	Page
Introduction	1
Types of Medical Reports	3
Model Report Forms	7
Transcribing the Material	23
Special Typing Rules	25
Punctuation	25
Capitalization	25
Numbers, Figures, & Abbreviations	26
Roots	29
Prefixes	31
Suffixes	33
Case A—Amy Allison	35
Definitions of Words, Phrases, and Abbreviations	37
Case B—Bruce Babbs	51
Definitions of Words, Phrases, and Abbreviations	53
Case C—Clarence Carroll	63
Definitions of Words, Phrases, and Abbreviations	65
Cassette Quiz No. 1	77
Case D—Dorothy Deland	79
Definitions of Words, Phrases, and Abbreviations	81
Written Quiz No. 1	95
Case E—Elaine Erenburg	97
Definitions of Words, Phrases, and Abbreviations	99
Cassette Quiz No. 2	109
Case F—Frank Forch	111
Definitions of Words, Phrases, and Abbreviations	113
Case G—Gary Goldstein	123
Definitions of Words, Phrases, and Abbreviations	125
Written Quiz No. 2	137
Case H—Helen Hernandez	139
Definitions of Words, Phrases, and Abbreviations	141
Case I—Izumi Ishida	151
Definitions of Words, Phrases, and Abbreviations	153
Written Quiz No. 3	167
Case J—John K. Jenkins	169
Definitions of Words, Phrases, and Abbreviations	171
Cassette Quiz No. 3	179
Appendix	
Plates I to XII	181-192
Index of Words, Phrases, and Abbreviations	193

INTRODUCTION

What You Can Expect

This text/workbook is an extensive approach to the language of medicine which means that you will encounter nearly 1,000 medical terms, most of which will likely be new to you. These 1,000 words were selected by analyzing medical records at four medical institutions through the use of a computer. The most frequently used words were then included in the medical reports that follow.

It is not the purpose of this course to teach you all that you can learn regarding medical terminology, as such a course would take several semesters of intensive study. Within a time frame of approximately 40 hours, this course will expose to you a broad base of medical terms, give you medical transcription practice, and provide experience working with the more common medical reports. You should learn the terms presented as well as possible and develop the skill of spelling the more familiar words from memory while listening to the recorded reports.

About Medical Terms

Medical terms appear to be long and awkward because they are made up of combinations of other words. When a word is broken down into the various elements, however, it becomes easier to understand and to pronounce. For example, "enterocolitis" (en-ter-o-ko-li′ tis) means a nonspecific inflammation of the intestines. The word is comprised of three elements—*entero* from the Greek "enteron" meaning intestine, *col* from the Greek "kolon" meaning the large intestine, and *itis* also from the Greek derivation meaning inflammation of.

These elements are found in a great number of medical terms. Actually, once you are able to recognize the elements of a medical term, the spelling and meaning of the word can be determined from the elements.

What You Do

You will be typing reports from ten individual case histories, such as might be encountered in a large metropolitan medical center. These reports are to be typed on forms provided for you. There is one form for each kind of report needed in a given case. If you need extra forms to complete a report, refer to those provided as Models and make extra copies on your typewriter unless directed otherwise by your instructor.

The types of cases presented are derived from actual files and are true to life and accurate in detail. The words and phrases used have been selected from carefully screening typical hospital records in a metropolitan area. In each case, you will type the dictated reports that are pertinent to that particular patient from the time of admission to the medical center to the time of discharge. Before typing the case reports, go through the word list provided for each case (1) to become familiar with the spelling and (2) to get in mind the meaning of the word.

What You Have to Work With

A brief resumé is presented for each case. This is to acquaint you with the patient's progress from one area to another within the hospital, as well as to clarify the various reports needed for that individual case. The text also contains forms on which the dictated reports may be typed.

There is a comprehensive list of words and phrases for each case which details all the medical terms to be learned in that case. Definitions are given for each word or phrase that is new, and they have been kept nontechnical and easy to understand. As a help in pronunciation and word recognition, the terms used in the case are dictated at the beginning of each case cassette. In addition, there is a word-pronouncing cassette with all the medical terms contained in this course recorded in alphabetical order.

TYPES OF MEDICAL REPORTS

There are seven basic reports used in this transcription course. They are History and Physical Examination (sometimes referred to as an H & P), X-ray Report, Operative Record, Pathology Report, Consultant's Report, Discharge Summary (sometimes referred to as a Clinical Resume), and Autopsy Report. An explanation and example of each type of report follows. The format of these reports will vary according to the hospital, clinic, or medical office involved. In a hospital, the responsibility for designing the format belongs to the hospital forms committee. The formats used here shouldn't be construed as the only "correct" forms, but those that are accepted for this course.

As you look through the explanations given for each type of report, you will want to compare the explanation for a particular term, line, or section with the Model Report Forms which follow these explanations, beginning on page 7.

History and Physical Examination

When a patient is admitted to the hospital for evaluation and treatment, the attending physician will prepare a medical history detailing the illness and complaint which prompted admission to the hospital. In addition to the patient's personal history, information pertaining to family background and family history is often included. A REVIEW OF SYSTEMS is also included. This is a survey of possible symptoms or historical facts relating to the patient's organ systems (for example, heart, lungs, abdomen). You will notice that many negative facts, such as "no cough or chest pain," are included in this review in order to point out the probable exclusion of certain diseases. Some dictated reports will be more comprehensive than others, and the style of dictation may vary depending on the dictating physician.

This is a common format for the History and Physical Exam:

CHIEF COMPLAINT: (The principal symptoms which prompted the patient to seek medical attention.)
HISTORY OF PRESENT ILLNESS: (The history or evolution of the present illness.)
PAST HISTORY: (Pertinent past medical and social history.)
FAMILY HISTORY:
REVIEW OF SYSTEMS: Under the REVIEW OF SYSTEMS, you will notice that subheadings are used for each organ system described or examined. Not every dictating physician will include all the organ systems described in this course. Some that are not pertinent to the particular case may be omitted. The subheadings for REVIEW OF SYSTEMS generally include:
HEAD AND NECK:
CARDIORESPIRATORY: (The heart and respiratory systems or lungs.)
GASTROINTESTINAL: (The digestive system.)
GENITOURINARY: (The urinary organs and the genitals.)
GYNECOLOGIC: (The obstetrical history, menstrual history, and female organs.)
NERVOUS SYSTEM:
MUSCULOSKELETAL: (The muscles and bones of the body.)
ENDOCRINE: (The glands of internal secretion, such as the thyroid gland, pancreas, and adrenal gland.)
PHYSICAL EXAMINATION: Similarly, the subheadings under PHYSICAL EXAMINATION may vary.

The following are representative:
GENERAL: (The vital signs of the patient—the blood pressure, pulse, temperature, and respirations.)
GENERAL APPEARANCE:
HEAD AND NECK:
THORAX AND LUNGS: (The chest cavity and the lungs.)
CARDIAC: (The examination of the heart.)
ABDOMEN:
GENITALIA: (The examination of the genitals or sexual organs.)
ANUS AND RECTUM:
EXTREMITIES: (The limbs.)
NEUROLOGICAL: (The nervous system.)
SKIN:

At the end of the History and Physical Exam the various diagnoses or working diagnoses are listed. A suspected or possible diagnosis will be prefaced by the words "rule out."

The History and Physical Examination report is a priority item in the hospital transcription room because it is the summary of the information known at the time of admission. It should be included with the patient's record on the hospital floor as soon as possible.

X-ray Report

The X-ray Report is a description of the findings and interpretations of the radiologist as he or she reviews X-rays done on a patient. The reports may be simply a description of plain X-rays taken of a certain part of the body, such as an X-ray of the wrist, or it may be a special study, such as a gastrointestinal series (GI), to evaluate the stomach and the bowels.

Various kinds of special studies will be included in this series of exercises to familiarize you with them. For example, newer techniques of examination of an organ by isotopes (radioactive material) are presented in X-ray Reports. These are called "scans."

The X-ray Report includes the preliminary information at the top of the report, the general type of X-ray examination done, followed by the IMPRESSION of the X-ray examination. Several different X-ray examinations of the patient may be included in the same report.

The results of an X-ray are typed immediately since it may affect immediate patient care.

Operative Record

The Operative Record includes the preoperative and postoperative diagnosis, the surgeon and assistants, the description of the operation, and the findings and procedures used in the operation. It is dictated within 24 hours of the completion of the operative procedure.

The body of the report is in narrative form. You will notice in the example of the Operative Record that the FINDINGS AND PROCEDURES are dictated and typed in one long paragraph. Although this may seem unwieldy to you, this is exactly how the great majority of surgeons dictate their operative records; that is, a running commentary without paragraphs. This is how they appear on most hospital charts.

Surgical suture material has its own description of size and is measured in gauges as follows: zero = 0 (strong and thick), five zero = 00000 (very thin), and so forth. Thus, if a surgeon dictates, "skin closed with three zero silk suture," this may be typed as, "skin closed with 000 silk suture" or "skin closed with 3-0 silk suture." The latter method is the one used in the model report forms. Very heavy suture material will be described in numerals, such as 1, 2, 3. For example, No. 1 silk suture.

Pathology Report

Pathology Reports are reports of tissue or fluid taken from the body which are examined by the pathologist to determine the nature and extent of the disease.

In a description of tissue examined, the pathologist will usually refer to a gross and microscopic description. The GROSS description is that of the tissue as it has been received in the laboratory and examined "grossly" or by the naked eye before it is prepared for microscopic study. The MICROSCOPIC description is that of the tissue after it has been prepared and carefully examined under the microscope.

Consultant's Report

If the admitting physician seeks the opinion or advice of a consultant, the consultant will write or dictate a Consultant's Report. The body of the report expresses the findings and views of the consultant.

Discharge Summary

The Discharge Summary is dictated by the physician upon the discharge of the patient from the hospital. The type of form may vary from hospital to hospital. It includes the date of admission, the date of discharge of the patient, the patient's diagnosis, surgery that has been performed, whatever complications ensued, and whatever special diagnostic procedures were carried out. Consultations, which were obtained from other physicians, are also recorded. This is followed by the body of the report which is dictated in narrative form by the physician. Sometimes the term Clinical Resumé is used instead of Discharge Summary.

Autopsy Report

The Autopsy Report, included in the last case of this course, includes a clinical history, which is a brief resumé of the patient's medical history and course in the hospital prior to demise, followed by the GROSS ANATOMY report, which is an examination of the patient before any tissues are removed for preparation and examination under the microscope. This is followed by the MICROSCOPIC EXAMINATION, which is an examination of the particular organs microscopically. The last part of the report is the actual findings listed as the FINAL PATHOLOGICAL DIAGNOSIS.

Model Report Forms

As you read through the Model Report Forms, you will notice that in all models, both the abbreviation and its meaning are included. This is not the case in medical transcripts. While hospital policy varies, the AMA recommends using the fully written out version rather than the abbreviation.

In the REVIEW OF SYSTEMS, a section of the History and Physical Exam, a particular organ system may be included in the subheadings and then described in one word as "Noncontributory." This means that there are no factors or symptoms referrable to that organ system pertinent to the case.

The vital signs referred to in the dictation of the History and Physical Exam under physical examination refer to the four basic signs of life; that is, blood pressure, pulse, temperature, and respirations.

The blood pressure is comprised of two numbers, systolic and diastolic. It is usually dictated, for example, as 120 over 80. It may be typed as such, but it is more commonly typed 120/80.

The pulse is dictated as the number of beats per minute and is typed, for example, as 80 per minute or 80/min.

The temperature is recorded either in degress Celsius (also called Centigrade) or Fahrenheit and is usually typed as 37°C or 98.6°F. Degrees Celsius will be used throughout the dictation in this course.

The respirations reflect the number of breaths per minute and is typed, for example, as 14 per minute or 14/min.

Model Report Form

Metropolitan Medical Center

HISTORY AND PHYSICAL EXAM

name Cynthia Freeze
address 2184 Airport Road
Belmont, MD 20860-4624

date June 8, 19--
physician Ann Marie Noyes, M.D.

hospital no. 436827
date of birth April 18, 19--
occupation Homemaker
race Caucasian
room no. 536

CHIEF COMPLAINT: Severe pain in the right side that radiates into the groin of approximately 8 hours' duration.

HISTORY OF PRESENT ILLNESS: The patient is a 39-year-old homemaker who awoke early this morning with severe pain in the right side associated with some nausea and vomiting. The pain has gotten gradually worse and seems to come in waves. She was taken to the hospital where initial evaluation with an intravenous pyelogram showed evidence of a right ureteral calculus in the midportion of the ureter with attendant Grade II hydronephrosis. The patient denies any associated hematuria, fever, chills, or dysuria.

PAST HISTORY: The patient is Gravida II, Para II, ab 0. She had an appendectomy done approximately 4 years ago and has generally been in good health since that time. She smokes approximately 10 cigarettes per day. Her periods have been normal without any dysmenorrhea or metrorrhagia.

FAMILY HISTORY: The patient's father is a diabetic who is treated by diet alone. The patient's mother died at age 48 of cancer of the breast.

REVIEW OF SYSTEMS:

HEAD AND NECK: The patient denies any diplopia, headache, or upper respiratory tract symptoms.

CARDIORESPIRATORY: There has been no cough or dyspnea.

GASTROINTESTINAL: As noted above, she has had some attendant nausea and vomiting, but her bowel habits have been normal.

GENITOURINARY: There is a colicky pain in the right side which began the morning of admission. No dysuria, hematuria, or frequency of urination.

GYNECOLOGIC: The patient denies any vaginal discharge or dysmenorrhea. There has been no vaginal spotting.

NERVOUS SYSTEM: There has been no dizziness, muscle weakness, vertigo, or ataxia.

MUSCULOSKELETAL: There have been no symptoms of muscle pain or joint swelling.

ENDOCRINE: Noncontributory.

PHYSICAL EXAMINATION:

GENERAL: Blood pressure 130/80, pulse 112 and regular, temperature 37.6°C orally, respirations 16 per minute.

GENERAL APPEARANCE: The patient appears pale and diaphoretic and appears to have difficulty lying still in bed.

HEAD AND NECK: The thyroid is normal. Funduscopic exam is negative. There are no cervical nodes, and the trachea is in the midline.

THORAX AND LUNGS: There is good expansion of the chest, and the lungs are normal to percussion and auscultation.

CARDIAC: There is normal sinus rhythm without any evidence of murmurs, thrills, or rales.

ABDOMEN: There is some muscle guarding in the right upper quadrant and right lower quadrant. The bowel sounds are quiet.

GENITALIA: The vagina is normal and there is no evidence of any vaginal discharge. Bimanual examination shows marked tenderness of the fallopian tubes bilaterally with thickening.

ANUS AND RECTUM: Normal.

EXTREMITIES: No evidence of any edema or joint swelling.

NEUROLOGICAL: The deep tendon reflexes are normal, and there are no pathological reflexes present.

SKIN: The skin is warm and moist to touch. No cutaneous lesions are identified.

PHYSICAL DIAGNOSIS: (1) Right ureteral calculus with obstruction.
(2) Rule out pelvic inflammatory disease.

Model Report Form

Metropolitan Medical Center

X-RAY REPORT

name	Harry Rhein	**hospital no.**	368425
age	44	**x-ray no.**	8432
sex	Male	**room no.**	418B
physician	Robert Miller, M.D.	**date**	June 8, 19--

Posteroanterior and lateral views of the chest show no evidence of any active disease. The lung fields are clear without any evidence of infiltration; the cardiac silhouette is of normal size. The bronchovascular markings are normal. There is some slight calcification of the aortic knob.

IMPRESSION: Normal chest X-ray.

EXAMINATION: IVP

The bones and soft tissue shadows are normal. The renal outlines are normal, and there is prompt excretion of contrast material bilaterally. There is normal architecture and no evidence of calculus or obstruction. There is no residual.

IMPRESSION: Normal IVP.

EXAMINATION: Lung scan

The scan shows uniform distribution bilaterally without areas of varying density.

IMPRESSION: Normal lung scan.

EXAMINATION: Barium enema

The contrast material fills the sigmoid and all of the large bowel normally. There are no areas of constriction.

IMPRESSION: Normal barium enema.

EXAMINATION: Upper gastrointestinal series

The esophagus, stomach, and duodenum fill out completely with normal emptying. No ulcers or tumors are seen.

IMPRESSION: Normal study.

Model Report Form

Metropolitan Medical Center

OPERATIVE RECORD

name	Richard Felter	**hospital no.**	68406
preoperative diagnosis	Left ureteral calculus	**room no.**	132A
postoperative diagnosis	Left ureteral calculus	**date**	June 18, 19--
surgeon	R. J. McCoy, M.D.	**first assistant**	Ronald Flint, M.D.
second assistant	None	**instrument nurse**	Arlene McDonald, R.N.
circulating nurse	Sarah Lawson, R.N.	**sponge count**	Correct

operation title or description Left ureterolithotomy (removal of calculus from left ureter)

FINDINGS AND PROCEDURES:

Under satisfactory general endotracheal anesthesia, the patient was prepped and draped in the supine position. A left lower quadrant incision was made through the skin and subcutaneous tissues to the external oblique fascia. This was opened and the underlying internal oblique muscle was split in the direction of the fibers. The underlying transversus muscle was also split and the transversalis fascia opened. The peritoneum was then retracted medially exposing the deep pelvic retroperitoneal area. The left ureter was identified and freed up by blunt and sharp dissection. The calculus was palpated within the ureter approximately 3 cm below the point where the ureter crosses the iliac artery. Clamps were applied to the ureter just above and below the calculus, and a longitudinal ureterotomy incision was made over the calculus. The calculus was extracted and the ureter explored above and below for further calculi. The clamps were removed and the incision closed with 4-0 chromic catgut sutures. A Penrose drain was placed in apposition to the incision in the ureter and brought out to the exterior through a separate stab wound in the muscle and skin. Retraction was released and all muscle layers were allowed to fall into close apposition. The transversalis fascia, transversus muscle, internal oblique muscle, and external oblique fascia were closed in separate layers with interrupted 0 chromic catgut sutures. The subcutaneous tissues were closed with interrupted 3-0 plain catgut and the skin with interrupted 4-0 silk. The drain was secured to the skin with a single suture of 0 silk. A sterile dressing was applied. The patient left the Operating Room in satisfactory condition.

Model Report Form

Metropolitan Medical Center
PATHOLOGY REPORT

name	Viola Morrison	**hospital no.**	462800
tissue	Needle biopsy of the kidney	**room no.**	216
date received	February 4, 19--	**pathology report no.**	25-7890
date reported	February 6, 19--		

GROSS: The tissue is submitted as a small cylindrical piece of pale tissue measuring 2 cm in length and approximately 2 mm in width. The tissue is reddish-yellow in appearance and firm in texture. The specimen is totally imbedded in paraffin for preparation.

MICROSCOPIC: Examination of several areas microscopically reveal normal renal architecture with normal glomeruli. The basement membranes are intact. There is some fibrosis about the tubular structures with interstitial infiltration with both leukocytes and lymphocytes. Some of the arterioles show some thickening of the wall.

PATHOLOGICAL DIAGNOSIS: Chronic pyelonephritis.

Model Report Form

Metropolitan Medical Center

CONSULTANT'S REPORT

to Dr. Abraham Bauman   **hospital no.** 268931

from Dr. Maria Balboa   **room no.** 218B

re Gordon Thomas   **date** August 4, 19—

reason for consultation Abdominal pain

    The patient's principal complaint is that of weakness, fatigue, and vague abdominal pain of several days' duration. He states that he has had some nausea, but there has been no vomiting, colic, or diarrhea. He has noted dark, tarry stools over the past 3 days. He has been afebrile and in spite of anorexia has been able to drink liquids and take some food.

    His past history is pertinent in that he had been treated for a duodenal ulcer 12 years ago but has been on no particular regimen since that time.

    On physical exam, there was some tenderness in the upper abdomen but no rebound. There was no organomegaly or mass palpable. A stool guaiac was positive. His hematocrit was 28 vols% and his hemoglobin 8.7 gm%.

    I feel that he has a recurrence of his duodenal ulcer with bleeding leading to his current condition of abdominal pain and weakness.

    I have arranged for an upper GI series and have placed him on an ulcer regimen. We will follow him directly with you. Thank you for your referral.

Model Report Form

Metropolitan Medical Center

DISCHARGE SUMMARY

name Faris Burns	**hospital no.** 468442
admitted January 15, 19--	**room no.** 618
discharged January 19, 19--	**age** 36
diagnosis Hiatal hernia	

surgery None

complications None

special procedures None

consultations None

Faris Burns was admitted for evaluation and treatment of sharp substernal chest pain which had been present for 3 days prior to admission on an intermittent basis. The pain was not associated with any shortness of breath, dyspnea, or physical exertion. He did complain of some mild burning in the stomach after eating. There had been no vomiting or hematemesis and no weakness, fatigue, or diaphoresis.

His past history is essentially negative. He has been in good health. He smokes 1 pack of cigarettes per day and has done so for 15 years. He had a routine prior physical examination 1 year ago including an EKG which was normal.

On physical examination, the chest was clear to percussion and auscultation. The cardiac exam was negative; there were no murmurs. The heart sounds were normal; there was no gallop. There was some mild epigastric tenderness to palpation. Bowel sounds were normal.

A complete blood count and urine were negative. An EKG was also normal without evidence of ischemia. A chest X-ray was negative. An upper GI series demonstrated a small sliding hiatal hernia.

He was placed on antacids and a bland diet and instructed to sleep with his head and chest slightly elevated on pillows.

He was discharged from the hospital on January 19 asymptomatic and is to be followed as an outpatient. He is to continue the regimen outlined above.

Model Report Form

Metropolitan Medical Center

AUTOPSY REPORT

name   Hector Moreno   **hospital no.**   864902

physician   Ardith Wightman, M.D.   **room no.**   322

pathology report no.   6842-2

CLINICAL HISTORY: The patient is a 38-year-old male with a long history of chronic renal failure secondary to chronic pyelonephritis. He had been on treatment for the past 3 years and was admitted at this time for further treatment because of the onset of congestive heart failure.

Subsequent to starting his hemodialysis, the patient developed gram negative infection and profound shock. He was started on the appropriate antibiotics and life-sustaining measures including intravenous cortisone.

His general condition deteriorated until he expired on the third hospital day from overwhelming infection.

Initial laboratory studies done on his admission showed a blood urea nitrogen of over 200 mg%. His white blood count was 3,800 with a normal differential. His hematocrit was 24 and his hemoglobin 6.2. An electrocardiogram showed evidence of left ventricular strain, and a chest X-ray showed evidence of pulmonary effusions bilaterally.

GROSS ANATOMY:

The body is that of a very thin male with poor muscle substance. The body measures 174.5 cm in length and weighs 54 kg. Rigor mortis is 2+, and liver mortis in the dependent parts of the body is noted. The head is normal and covered by black hair. The sclerae are pale and irides are brown. The pupils are equal. The teeth are in good repair. The chest is symmetrical and the abdomen is mildly protuberant. The external genitalia are normal. The extremities reveal 2+ edema of the ankles and feet.

NECK ORGANS: The trachea is in proper position, and there are no abnormal lymph nodes or tumors.

THORAX: The pleural spaces are filled with frothy opaque fluid. The lungs are pink and appear normal. The organ relationship is not disturbed.

ABDOMEN: The peritoneum is thin, and there is approximately 600 cc of fluid removed from the abdominal cavity. The surfaces of the intestines are dusky and bluish in color. The mesenteric vessels are markedly engorged.

RESPIRATORY SYSTEM: The right lung weighs 400 gm and the left lung 600 gm. They are firm in texture and there appears to be a normal bronchovascular relationship.

CARDIOVASCULAR SYSTEM: The heart weighs 400 gm. The left ventricle is markedly enlarged and dilated. There is a vegetative growth on the aortic valve. There is some scarring noted in the mitral valve area. The coronary arteries are normal.

GASTROINTESTINAL SYSTEM: The intestines appear to be somewhat edematous and dusky in color. The mesenteric vessels are dilated and engorged.

LIVER: The liver weighs 1800 gm and the surface is smooth. There is no evidence of any fibrosis and a cut surface appears normal.

PANCREAS: The pancreas appears normal without any evidence of fibrosis or nodules.

GENITOURINARY SYSTEM: The kidneys each weigh 80 gm. The capsules are firmly adherent and there is marked pitting noted. There is severe atrophy of the cortex. There appears to be focal areas of fibrosis throughout the kidneys. The urinary bladder appears normal. The prostate is unremarkable.

ENDOCRINE: The thyroid and adrenals are normal without any evidence of nodularity or atrophy.

BRAIN: The brain weighs 1500 gm. On sectioning, normal relationship of gray matter to white matter is noted. The vascularity appears normal. There is no evidence of any edema.

MICROSCOPIC EXAMINATION:

HEART: There is marked attenuation and thinness of the myocardium of the left ventricle. The muscle bundles are generally uniform. There is marked fibrosis and distortion with an infiltration of leukocytes in the valvular areas.

LUNGS: Several sections reveal normal aveoli with normal bronchovascular relationships and no evidence of infiltration.

LIVER: The hepatic architecture appears normal with normal portal areas. There is no evidence of any interstitial inflammation nor evidence of cholestasis.

KIDNEYS: There is marked atrophy and decrease in numbers of the glomeruli and tubules. The vessels appear to be thickened with obliteration of the lumens of the arterioles. There is a chronic inflammatory infiltrate of leukocytes in the interstitial tissue between the tubules. The ducts appear to be somewhat congested. There is marked fibrosis of the basement membranes of the glomeruli.

PROSTATE: The prostate is normal in size with normal architecture and no evidence of carcinoma.

FINAL PATHOLOGICAL DIAGNOSIS:

RESPIRATORY SYSTEM: Bilateral pleural effusion.

CARDIOVASCULAR: Bacterial endocarditis.

GASTROINTESTINAL TRACT: Mesenteric vein thrombosis with passive congestion of the small bowel.

GENITOURINARY: Chronic pyelonephritis.

ENDOCRINE: No evidence of thyroid or adrenal disease.

MUSCULOSKELETAL: Marked pedal and ankle edema present.

CAUSE OF DEATH: Renal failure secondary to chronic pyelonephritis with attendant congestive heart failure.

TRANSCRIBING THE MATERIAL

By transcribing the dictated material on these various reports as each pertains to the individual case history, you will become familiar with the many varied hospital procedures and the broad range of medical vocabulary. A new word will be listed and defined in "Definitions of Words, Phrases, and Abbreviations" when it first appears in a case report. When the word is used in subsequent cases and you cannot remember its meaning, refer to the alphabetical word list in the Appendix. You will find there what word list to refer to for the meaning of the word.

It is suggested that you listen to an entire case on cassette while studying the word list from that particular case. Stop and start the cassette as often as desired. In this way, you can familiarize yourself with the pronunciation and the meaning of the various words. After you have done this, go back to the beginning of the dictation and start your transcription. You should listen to several words or phrases at a time, then stop and type. If it is not fully understood, go back and listen. When it is clear, begin your typing.

Before beginning your transcription, review the appropriate Model Report Forms. It would be wise, too, to study the list of common prefixes and suffixes used in medical terminology. Also included is a brief description of the roots used for the derivation of many medical words.

There are also anatomical plates for you to view and examine prior to and during the transcription of the medical case histories. These plates are located in the Appendix. The plates related to each case are listed in the introduction to the case.

Through this procedure and with time and practice, you will develop some facility for picking up the meaning of words and the general structure and content of the sentences used in medical reports.

Also carefully review the following general considerations before beginning your transcription:

(1) The definition given in the word list for the terms and phrases used will not necessarily be comprehensive or include all of the possible meanings for that term. Rather, the meaning given will be brief and pertinent to the context of that particular exercise. The medical dictionary should be consulted as much as possible to fully familiarize yourself with the words and concepts.

(2) Standard abbreviations for medical terms, if used by the dictating physician, may be used in the transcription. Some common abbreviations are listed on page 28.

(3) The names of drugs used in the dictation will generally be trade names rather than generic (or chemical) names.

(4) In the subheadings of the various reports, capital letters are used. The Model Report Forms should be followed as a guide.

(5) Some medical terms are spelled the same but have slightly different meanings depending on the context in which they are used. For example, "infiltrate" used as a noun means the influx of cells or tissues into an area. "Infiltrate" used as a verb has the accent on the second syllable and means to introduce or cause the influx of fluid or medication into an area.

When you have completed your transcription, fill in the date under that particular report in the "Sequence of Reports" on the first page of the Case.

Each case history is designed to take approximately four hours. The actual time will depend on your background, aptitude, and preparation. It is not to be assumed that the terms will be throughly learned within that time frame.

SPECIAL TYPING RULES

There are some special rules that apply to typing medical information. This section contains some of the punctuation, capitalization, number, abbreviation, figure, and symbol rules that you should know and use in the transcription of medical data.

Punctuation

Rule 1. Use a hyphen when two or more words are viewed as a single word.

Example: On follow-up examination, the symptoms were no longer present.

She is a well-developed, well-nourished Caucasian female.

Rule 2. Use a hyphen when words are compounded with figures.

Example: He is a 35-year-old salesman in no acute distress.

Capitalization

Rule 3. Capitalize eponyms. Eponyms are surnames teamed with a disease, instrument, or surgical procedure. The American Medical Association recommends that an eponym not be used if a comparable medical term is available.

Example: Romberg's sign
Foley catheter
Kelly clamps

Rule 4. Capitalize trade names (including trademarked suture materials) and brand names of drugs and trademarked material. Generic drugs and suture materials are not capitalized.

Example: Trade names of drugs
Keflex, Coumadin

Trade names of suture materials
Dermalon

Generic names of drugs
potassium, alcohol

Generic names of suture materials
catgut, nylon, cotton

Rule 5. Capitalize nouns that immediately precede numbers or letters.

Example: Gravida II, Para II
Grade II systolic murmur

Rule 6. Capitalize the names of specific departments or sections of the hospital.

Example: Intensive Care, Admitting Office, Emergency Room

Rule 7. Capitalize the names of the genus, but not the names of the species that often follow it. The genus may be referred to by its first initial only (capitalized, with a period following it, and then the species name).

Example: E. coli (Escherichia coli)

Numbers, Figures, and Abbreviations

Rule 8. Spell out ordinal numbers indicating order or succession.

    Example: There was trauma to the fifth and sixth ribs.

                  On the third day of hospitalization, a heart catheterization was performed.

Rule 9. Use figures in writing age, weight, height, blood pressure, pulse, respiration, dosage, size, and temperature.

    Example: This is a 26-year-old, well-developed, well-nourished, white female. Height: 165 cm. Weight: 56.8 kg. Blood Pressure: 120/80. Pulse: 72. Respirations: 18/min.

Rule 10. Where numbers would traditionally be typed slightly above or below the line as superscript or subscript, current practice is to type them on the line, except when power is indicated (10^3).

    Example: H_2O type H2O
                A_2 type A2
                L_4 type L4

Rule 11. Use figures when numbers are used directly with symbols, words, or abbreviations.

    Example: 3%
                1+ protein

Rule 12. Use figures when writing suture materials.

    Example: 3-0 or 000

Rule 13. Use figures with capital letters to refer to the vertebral column.

    Example: The disk was herniated at L4-5.

Rule 14. Use figures when writing electrocardiographic leads.

    Example: The intrinsicord deflection was 0.08 sec. in V6.

Rule 15. Use figures and symbols when writing plus or minus with a number.

    Example: 1+ to 2+

Roman Numerals

Rule 16. Roman numerals are used in the following situation.

Class	Class III malignancy
Cranial leads (EKG)	Lead I reading
Cranial nerves	Cranial nerve V and VI
Factor (blood clotting)	Factor V
Grade	Grade II systolic murmur
Phase	Phase II clinical trials
Pregnancy and delivery	Gravida II Para II
Stage	Stage I carcinoma
Type	Type I

Abbreviations

Rule 17. Use abbreviations for all metric measurements used with numbers. Type metric measures in the lowercase, one space after the number. They are not made plural. Celsius and Fahrenheit (C and F) are exceptions. Punctuation may be omitted.

    Example: 2 mm
                    37°C

Rule 18. Chemical and mathematic abbreviations are written in a combination of both upper and lowercase letters without periods.

Example:	Hgb	hemoglobin
	Hg	mercury
	Na	sodium
	T4	thyroxine
	NaCl	sodium chloride
	K	potassium

Rule 19. Units of measurement are typed in lowercase letters without periods.

    Example: cm, in, cc, ft, gr, mm, oz

Rule 20. Latin abbreviations are typed in lowercase letters with periods.

Example:	b.i.d.	twice a day
	t.i.d.	three times a day
	q.i.d.	four times a day
	a.c.	before meals

Metric Measures

The metric system of measurements is used in medicine. Laboratory determinations are expressed in grams, kilograms, milligrams, and micrograms. Fluid measurements are in liters and milliliters, volumes in cubic centimeters, and lengths in meters and centimeters. A standard medical dictionary will include a comprehensive list of metric measurements and their abbreviations.

When typing numbers with metric measurements use abbreviations. Punctuation is not used with metric abbreviations.

Here is a list of some common abbreviations used:

gram(s)	gm
kilogram(s)	kg (not kilo)
milligram(s)	mg
microgram(s)	mcg
centimeter(s)	cm
cubic centimeter(s)	cc
millimeter(s)	mm
liter(s)	L or *l*

Laboratory Test Results

Laboratory test results using metric measures are reported with abbreviations. Those used in this text include:

volume percent	vols%
grams percent	gm%
milligrams percent	mg%
cubic millimeter	cc mm

Names of tests are often reported using abbreviations. Some examples used in this course include:

CBC	complete blood count
LDH	lactic dehydrogenase
pCO_2	partial pressure of carbon dioxide
pO_2	partial pressure of oxygen
RBC	red blood cell
SGOT	serum glutamic-oxalactic transaminase
SGPT	serum glutamic-pyruoic transaminase
WBC	white blood cell

Other Abbreviations Used

Additional abbreviations which follow are used in the cases in this course. These abbreviations pertinent to this course may be used, but only if you fully understand them.

ab	abortio
AP	anteroposterior
BP	blood pressure
BPH	benign prostatic hypertrophy
D & C	dilation and currettage
DTR	deep tendon reflex
E. coli	Escherichia coli
EKG	electrocardiogram
ER	emergency room
GI	gastrointestinal
ICU	intensive care unit
IPPB	intermittent positive pressure breathing
IVP	intravenous pyelogram
JVP	jugular venous pulse
L3, L4	third and fourth lumbar vertebrae
poly	polymorphonuclear leukocyte
PA	posteroanterior
Para	successful term pregnancies
PMI	point of maximum impulse
PTA	prior to admission
T and A	tonsillectomy and adenoidectomy
T_{11}	thoracic vertebra
WNL	within normal limits

There is one place in which abbreviations are considered unacceptable, according to the Joint Commission of Accreditation of Hospitals. This is on the front sheet attached to the discharge summary. This is the sheet that hospital coding utilizes, and all terms must be written in full.

ROOTS

A root is that element of a word which is neither prefix nor suffix. It is the word element denoting the origin of a word and in medicine frequently refers to a part of the body or bodily function. It may appear in the first part of a word such as *broncho*gram. It may have a prefix or a suffix attached or both as extra*bronch*ial. Words may also have more than one root.

The following list is certainly not comprehensive but will serve as a basic guideline of many roots you will come across in this course and in the typing of subsequent medical reports. You can guess at the meaning of many words by studying this and similar lists of medical word roots.

A

ADEN(o)—gland
adenopathy—diseased gland
ANGI(o)—vessel
angiography—X-ray of blood vessels
ARTER(i)—artery
arteriosclerosis—hardening of arteries
ARTHR(o)—joint
arthrotomy—incision into a joint

B

BRACHI(o)—arm
brachiocephalic—pertaining to the arm and head
BRONCH(o)—bronchus, windpipe
bronchovascular—involving bronchi and blood vessels
BUCC(o)—cheek
buccolabial—pertaining to the cheek and lips

C

CARCIN(o)—crab
carcinogenesis—the origin of cancer (the crab)
CARDI(o)—heart
cardiogenic—originating from the heart
CEPHAL(o)—head
cephalodynia—pain in the head
CEREBR(o)—cerebrum, brain
cerebromeningitis—inflammation of the brain and its membranes
CERVIC(o)—neck
cervicofacial—pertaining to the face and neck
CHOLE—bile
cholelith—biliary calculus (stone)
CHONDR(o)—cartilage
chondromalacia—a disease of cartilage causing it to become soft
COST(o)—rib
costochondral—pertaining to a rib and its cartilage

CRANI(o)—skull
craniocervical—pertaining to the skull and the neck
CYST(o)—bladder
cystoscope—instrument used to view the bladder
CYT(o)—cell
cytotoxic—harmful to cells

D

DERM(o)—skin
dermoplasty—skin grafting

E

ENTER(o)—intestine
enterocolitis—inflammation of the large intestine

G

GASTR(o)—stomach
gastroscope—instrument to view the stomach
GLOSS(o)—tongue
glossopharyngeal—pertaining to the tongue and pharynx

H

HEM(o)—blood
hemostasis—referring to the cessation of bleeding
HEPAT(o)—liver
hepatomegaly—enlargement of the liver
HYSTER(o)—uterus
hysterotomy—an incision into the uterus

I

ILE(o)—ileum (part of small bowel)
ileocecal—pertaining to the ileum and the cecum
ILI(o)—ilium (a bone in the pelvis)
iliosacral—pertaining to the ilium and sacrum

L

LABI(o)—lip
labioplasty—plastic surgery of the lip
LARYNG(o)—larynx
laryngoscope—an instrument to view the larynx
LIP(o)—fat
lipoma—a fatty tissue tumor

M

MAST(o)—breast
mastopathy—disease of the breast
MY(o)—muscle
myocardial—referring to the heart muscle
MYEL(o)—marrow—in specific reference it denotes the spinal cord
myelogram—X-ray of the spinal cord

N

NEPHR(o)—kidney
nephrosclerosis—hardening of the kidney
NEUR(o)—nerve
neurogenic—arising from the nerves

O

OPTHALM(o)—eye
opthalmoscopic—pertaining to an examination of the eye.
ORCHI(o)—testicle, testis
orchiopexy—surgical fixation of a testis

OSTE(o)—bone
osteomyelitis—inflammation of the bone and bone marrow
OT(o)—ear
otoplasty—plastic surgery of the ear
OV(o)—egg, ova
ovogenesis—the origin and development of the egg

P

PATH(o)—disease pathology—the study of disease and disease processes
PHLEB(o)—vein
phlebothrombosis—a blood clot within a vein
PNEUM(o)—air
pneumothorax—the accumulation of air or gas in the thoracic cavity
PROCT(o)—rectum
proctoscope—an instrument for viewing the rectum

PSYCH(o)—soul, mind
psychology—the study of human personality and development
PY(o)—pus
pyogenic—producing pus
PYEL(o)—pelvis
pyelonephritis—inflammation of the kidney and its pelvis

R

RADI(o)—ray
radiology—the study of X-rays
RHIN(o)—nose
rhinoplasty—plastic surgery of the nose

S

SALPING(o)—tube
salpingotomy—incision into the fallopian tube
STOM—mouth
stomatology—the study of diseases of the mouth

T

THORAC(o)—chest
thoraco-abdominal—referring to the chest and abdomen
TRACHE(o)—windpipe
tracheotomy—incision into the trachea

U

UR(o)—urine
urochrome—the yellow pigment in urine

PREFIXES

A prefix is one or more letters or syllables placed before a word to modify its meaning, such as, avascular (meaning without blood vessels or blood supply). Some words may have more than one prefix. This list is representative of prefixes used in this course, and their study can give you further insight into the development of a medical term.

A-, AN—without, lack of (*a* is used before consonants, *an* before vowels)
atonic—without tone; anemia—without blood
AB—away from
aberrant—wandering from or deviating away from the normal
AD—to, toward
adhesive—sticking to or clinging closely to
AMBI—both, on both sides
ambilateral—affecting both sides
ANTE—before
antecubital—situated in front of or before the cubitus (forearm)
ANTI—against, opposed to
antiemetic—a drug used against emesis or vomiting
ATEL—imperfect, incomplete
atelectasis—imperfect expansion of lungs at birth; collapse of adult lung

BI-, BIS—two, twice
bilobular—having two lobes
BRADY—slow
bradycardia—slow heart action

CATA—down, under, lower
cataphoria—a downward turning of the visual axes of the eyes
CIRCUM—around, about
circumflex—bent around, bent like a bow
CO-, COL-, CON—with, together
coexist—to exist together; confluence—a coming together
CONTRA—against, opposite
contraceptive—against conception
CRYPTO—hidden
cryptorchid—a hidden or undescended testicle

DE—down, away from

decompression—removal of pressure away from an organ or tissue
DEXTRO—right
dextrocardia—abnormality where the heart is on the right side of the thorax
DI—two, twice, double
diarthric—pertaining to two joints
DIS—reversal, separation
disacidify—to remove acid from
DYS—difficult, painful
dysmenorrhea—painful and difficult menstruation

EC-, ECTO-, EX-, EXO—out, outside, away from
ectopic—out of normal place
ENDO—within, inside
endocrine—secreting within or internally
EPI—on, upon
episcleral—overlying the sclerae
EXTRA—outside of, beyond, in addition to
extraocular—outside of the eye

HEMI—one half
hemiatrophy—atrophy (wasting) of one half of the body or of an organ
HOMEO—similar, same
homeostasis—a tendency toward uniformity or stability of the bodily functions
HYPER—above, over, excessive
hypertension—abnormally high tension, especially high blood pressure
HYPO—lack, deficiency
hypoactive—having a lack of activity

IM-, IN—into, in, on
impregnate—to render pregnant
IM-, IN—not
incurable—not able to be cured
INFRA—below

infravesicle—situated below the bladder
INTER—between
interdental—between the teeth
INTRA—within
intraductal—within a duct
INTRO—into, within
intromission—the insertion of one part into another

JUXTA—near, by
juxtaspinal—next to the spinal cord

LEUCO-, LEUKO—white
leukocyte—white blood cell

MEGA-, MAGALO—great, enlarged, large
megakayocyte—a large cell in the bone marrow
MESO—middle, moderate
mesoderm—the middle layer of the three primary germ layers of the embryo
META—between, after; or change, transformation
metacarpus—the part of the hand between the wrist and finger:
metaplasia—a change or transformation in the structure and composition of a cell

OB—against, in front of
obstruction—the act of blocking or clogging
ORTHO—straight, normal
orthochromatic—normally colored or stained

PARA—beside, beyond, accessory to
paradental—next to or alongside a tooth

PER—through, excessive
peracute—excessively acute or short
PERI—around
perirenal—around the kidney
POST—after, behind
postpartum—after delivery or childbirth
PRO—forward, before
prognosis—a forecast as to the probable result of a disease

RE—back, again, contrary
reinfect—to infect again

RETRO—backward, behind
retrograde—going backward, retracing a former course

SEMI—half, part of
semisupine—partly but not completely supine
SINISTRO—left
sinistromanual—left handed
STENO—narrow, contracted
stenostomia—narrowing of the mouth
SUB-, SUP—under, moderately
submandibular—below the jaw or mandible
SUPER—above, in excess of, over
supernumerary—in excess of the normal number
SUPRA—above, over
supraorbital—above the orbit (eye)
SYN—together with
syndrome—a set of symptoms which occur together

THERM-, THERMO—heat
thermography—the measurement of heat variations by a special device
TOX, TOXI—poison
toxigenic—capable of producing poisons
TRANS—across, through
transilluminate—to shine a light through

UNI—one
unilateral—affecting one side

SUFFIXES

A suffix is one or more syllables occurring at the end of the root or basic part of a term to modify its meaning. A medical term may have more than one suffix. Thus a word root is modified into a number of meanings; for example, pathology, derived from the root *(patho)* meaning disease or a diseased state and *(logy)* meaning the study of. We can therefore more easily understand words such as psych*ology*, cardi*ology*, neur*ology*.

-ALGIA—pain
cephalalgia—headache

-CELE—hernia, tumor, swelling
cystocele—a downward protrusion or hernia of the bladder

-CENTESIS—puncture, aspiration
culdocentesis—aspiration of fluid from the space between the uterus and rectum

-CLASIS—to break, destroy
osteoclasis—the surgical fracture or refracture of a bone

-CYTE—a hollow vessel, a cell
leukocyte—white blood cell

-ECTOMY—excision, cutting out
salpingectomy—excision of the salpinx (the fallopian tube)

-EMIA—blood condition
anemia—a condition reflecting the lack of blood

-GRAPH, -GRAPHY—writing or recording
cardiography—the recording of the heart's actions

-IASIS—state, condition of
cholelithiasis—the presence or state of having gallstones

-ITIS—inflammation
mastoiditis—inflammation of the mastoid sinus or process

-LOGY—the science or study of
pathology—the study of disease and disease processes

-LYSIS—to free, loosen
fibrinolysis—the dissolution of fibrin, a blood clotting element

-OID—like, similar
polypoid—polyp like in shape

-OMA—indicating a morbid condition, especially a tumor
adenoma—a benign glandular tumor

-OSIS—a disease condition or disease process
cirrhosis—a destructive disease of the liver

-PATHY—a state of illness or disease
adenopathy—disease of the lymph glands

-PEXY—surgical fixation
orchidopexy—fixation of an undescended testis into the scrotum

-PLASTY—repair
pyeloplasty—a repair of the kidney pelvis

-RRHAGE—profuse flow, a breaking or bursting forth
hemorrhage—a copious escape of blood from the vessels (bleeding)

-RRHAPHY—suture of
herniorrhapy—suture of, closure, and repair of a hernia

-RRHEA—flow
diarrhea—profuse flow of loose stool

-STOMY—creating an opening into or between
colostomy—the production of an artificial opening into the colon

-TAXIS—order, arrangement
chemotaxis—the phenomenon shown by certain cells of moving to or away from a chemical stimulus according to a certain order

-TOMY—cutting or incision
arthrotomy—incision into a joint

-TROPHIC—relating to nourishment or nutrition
hypertrophic—marked by a morbid enlargement or overgrowth of an organ

CASE A

Student: VANESSA

name Amy Allison

address 3704 Del Mar
San Diego, CA 92106-1321

situation This 29-year-old female suffering severe abdominal cramps, nausea, and vomiting was rushed to the medical center emergency room on January 15, 19—. Here she was examined and admitted to the hospital with a tentative diagnosis of appendicitis. She received blood studies and X-rays; then she was taken to surgery. An acutely inflamed appendix was removed and her convalescence was uneventful. She was discharged one week after admission.

When it was determined that the patient required surgery, a surgeon performed the appendectomy. In this situation, a general surgeon was involved. A surgeon may specialize in a particular branch of medicine or may operate for a variety of conditions, as in the case of general surgery.

Plate II in the Appendix relates to this case.

sequence of reports

A-1
History and Physical Exam
Completed _____

A-2
X-ray Report
Completed _____

A-3
Operative Record
Completed _____

A-4
Pathology Report
Completed _____

A-5
Discharge Summary
Completed _____

Note: Enter the date of completion for each report. When you have finished all the reports, tear this sheet out and give to your instructor along with the completed transcripts.

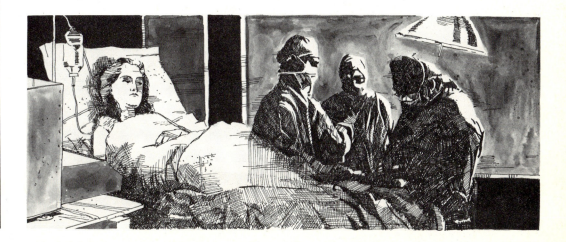

DEFINITIONS OF WORDS, PHRASES, AND ABBREVIATIONS

The following words, phrases, and abbreviations are used in Case A. Preview the words carefully and listen to the pronunciation of each on the tapes. Remember, correct transcript of the doctor's dictation is critical. Study the spelling with that thought in mind.

A

abortio (ab) (a-bor'shi-o)—number of aborted pregnancies.
abscess (ab'ses)—a pus pocket—an area of accumulation of pus.
accommodation (ah-kom-o-da'-shun)—ability to adjust from near vision to far.
adenitis (ad-eh-ni'tis)—inflammation of the lymph glands.
adenopathy (ad-e-nop'ah-the)—enlarged lymph glands.
adnexa (ad-nek'sa)—the ovaries and tubes (part of the female reproductive tract).
anesthesia (an-es-the'ze-ah)—loss of sensation or feeling of pain.
anorexia (an-o-rek'se-ah)—lack of appetite.
appendiceal (ap-pen-dis-e'al)—referring to the appendix.
appendicitis (ah-pen-di-si'tis)—inflammation of the appendix.
appendix (ah-pen'diks)—an accessory finger-like projection of bowel tissue arising from the cecum. (See Plate II, Appendix.)
auscultation (aws-kul-ta'shun)—listening to the sounds of breathing or the heart using a stethoscope.

B

Babinski (bah-bin'ske)—a neurological test or sign (Babinski's reflex).
band neutrophil (nu'tro-fil)—an immature neutrophil, the percentage of which are increased in acute bacterial infections.
Bartholin's gland (bar'to-linz)—a gland in the female genitalia.
basophil (ba'so-fil)—a type of white blood cell which is the least abundant in number.
bile (bil)—a yellowish-green digestive fluid produced by the liver.
BP—blood pressure

C

calculus (kal'ku-lus): plural, **calculi** (kal'ku-li)—stone.
cardiac (kar'de-ak)—pertaining to the heart.
cardiomegaly (kar-de-o-me'gale)—enlargement of the heart.
cardiorespiratory (kar-de-o-res'pir-ah-to-re)—pertaining to the heart and respiratory passages.
CBC—complete blood count
cecum (se'kum)—the very first part of the large bowel. (See Plate II, Appendix.)
cervical (ser've-kal)—referring to a neck.
cervix (ser'viks)—the neck of the womb. (See Plate X, Appendix.)
chromic catgut (kro'mik)—a type of dissolving suture with special strength.
claudication (klaw-de-ka'shun)—muscular cramps, usually brought on by exercise.
colic (kol'ik)—sharp, severe, intermittent pain.
colicky (kol'ik-e)—affected by colic.
convalescence (kon-vah-les'ens)—the stage of recovery after surgery or disease.
costovertebral angle (kos-to-ver-te'bral)—the angle made where a rib joins the vertebra in the back.
cranial (kra'ne-al)—pertaining to the head or cranium.
cylindrical (sil-in'dre-kl)—having the shape of a cylinder (a solid body shaped like a column).

D

deep tendon reflex (DTR)—the response to stimulation of a tendon by striking it.
diabetes (di-ah-be'tez)—a disease of having too much sugar in the blood.
diaphragm (di'ah-fram)—the muscular partitions between the thoracic and the abdominal cavity.
diastolic (di-ah-stol'ik)—the lower number of the blood pressure.
dyspnea (disp'ne-ah)—difficult breathing.
dysuria (dis-u're-ah)—painful urination.

E

edema (e-de'mah)—swelling
electrolyte (e-lek'tro-lit)—the blood electrolyte or electrolytes which are sodium, potassium, chloride, and carbon dioxide.
endotracheal (en-do-tra'ke-al)—refers to anesthetic gasses passed directly into the trachea (windpipe).
eosinophil (e-o-sin'o-fil)—white blood cells which are few in number.
ER—emergency room
excise (ek-siz'); past tense, **excised** (ek-sizd)—to cut off or cut out.
external oblique muscle—a superficial muscle of the abdominal wall.
exudate (eks'u-dat)—a film of tissue fluid made of pus which may cover an infected organ.
exudative (eks'u-da-tiv)—pertaining to or having an exudate.

F

fascia (fash'e-ah)—a sheet of fibrous tissue which envelops the body beneath the skin, and also encloses the muscles and groups of muscles and separates their several layers or groups.
focal (fo'kal)—appearing in a limited specific area or areas.
funduscopic exam (fun-dus-ko'pik)—examination of the fundus (innermost part) of the eye.

G

gallop—an abnormal rate and sound of the heartbeat.
gastrointestinal (GI) (gas-tro-in-tes'tin-al)—the digestive system (the stomach and bowels).
general anesthesia (an-es-the'ze-ah)—an anesthetic whereby the patient is put to sleep and totally anesthetized.
Gravida (grav'id-ah)—number of pregnancies.

gynecologic (gin-e-ko-lo'jik)—referring to the female genital organs.

H

hematemesis (hem-at-em'e-sis)—vomiting of blood.
hematocrit (hem-ah'to-krit)—a blood test representing the percentage of red blood cells in the blood by volume.
hematuria (hem-ah-tu're-ah)—blood in the urine.
hemoglobin (he-mo-glo'bin)—a blood test denoting the amount of oxygen carrying material in the blood stream and thus a parallel estimation of the amount of red blood cells in the blood.
hemorrhage (hem'or-ij)—bleeding or blood loss.
hemostasis (he-mos-tah'sis)—a stoppage of bleeding or adequate control of bleeding.

I

ileocecal junction (il-e-o-se'kal)—an anatomical landmark where the ileum joins the cecum.
ileum (il'e-um)—the very last part of the small bowel. (See Plate II, Appendix.)
infiltration (in-fil-tra'shun)—an ingrowth or influx of cells or tissue into an area.
injected (in-jekt'ed)—denotes an increase in the amount of visible blood vessels.
internal oblique muscle—the muscle under the external oblique.
intestine (in-tes'tin)—the bowel, the digestive tube. (See Plate II, Appendix.)

J

jaundice (jawn'dis)—yellow discoloration of the skin or sclerae.

K

Kelly clamp—a type of crushing clamp developed by Dr. Kelly to secure or interrupt blood vessels.

L

lesion (le'zhun)—abnormal finding, such as a growth or shadow.
leukocyte (lu'ko-sit)—a white blood cell of which certain numbers appear in the blood.
leukocytosis (lu-ko-si-to'sis)—an abnormally large number of white blood cells appearing in the blood.
ligate (li'gat)—tie off.
ligatures (lig'a-churs)—a thread or material used to tie off tissue or blood vessels.
lymphocyte (lim'fo-sit)—a type of white blood cell which is less abundant than neutrophils.

M

McBurney incision—an incision in the right lower abdomen developed by Dr. McBurney especially for appendectomies.
membrane (mem'bran)—a lining on the inside or outside of an organ by a thin layer of tissue.
mesenteric (mes-en-ter'ik)—refers to the supportive structure or tether of the bowel.
mesoappendix (mes-o-ah-pen'diks)—the thin connective tissue attaching the appendix to the bowel containing the blood vessels to the appendix.
midline—the anatomic midpoint of the body or of an organ.
murmur (mur'mur)—abnormal heart sound.
muscle guarding—denotes involuntary tightening of the abdominal muscles over an area of tenderness and inflammation as a protective reflex.

N

neutrophil (nu'tro-fil)—the most predominant type of white blood cells which are increased in bacterial infection.
nocturia (nok-tu're-ah)—excessive voiding at night.
normocephalic (nor-mo-se-fal'ik)—having a normal shaped head.

O

orally (o'ral-le)—pertaining to the mouth.
organomegaly (or-gan-o-me'ga-le)—enlargement of any organ.

P

Para (par'ah)—successful term pregnancies.
percussion (per-kush'un)—evaluating the sounds produced by tapping on a part of the body such as the chest.
peritoneal (per-i-to-ne'al)—referring to the peritoneum.
peritoneum (per-i-to-ne'um)—the thin tissue envelope that contains the abdominal organs located below the protective abdominal muscles.
phenol (fe'nol)—a chemical caustic agent.
postoperative—the period of time after surgery.
prepped—the procedure whereby the surgical site is shaved (if necessary) and cleansed by an antiseptic immediately before surgery.
PTA—prior to admission
pubic bone (pu'bik)—the bone forming the front lower part of the pelvis just above the genital organs.
pulmonary (pul'mo-na-re)—referring to the lungs.

Q

quadrant (kwod'rant)—the anatomical division of the abdominal wall into four quadrants with the belly button as the center—the right upper quadrant, the right lower quadrant, the left upper quadrant, and the left lower quadrant.

R

radiation of pain—pain which extends or travels from one point on the body to another.
rebound tenderness—pain and tenderness elicited in the abdominal area upon the sudden release of

gentle compression placed on the abdomen by the examiner's hand.

renal (re'nal)—pertaining to the kidney.

respiration (res-pi-ra'shun)—the act of breathing.

respiratory (re-spir'ah-to-re)—referring to the breathing apparatus (nose, mouth, throat, lungs).

rhinitis (ri-ni'tis)—a cold in the nose.

rubella (roo-bel'ah)—German measles.

S

Scarlet fever—an infectious disease causing a rash.

sclerae (skle'ra)—the whites of the eyes. (See Plate V, Appendix.)

segmented neutrophil (nu'tro-fil)—a fully developed or mature neutrophil.

serosa (se-ro'sah)—the thin outermost connective tissue lining of a tubular hollow organ, such as the bowel—in this case the cecum.

serosal (se-ro'sal)—pertaining to the serosa.

serum (se'rum)—that portion of the blood tissue remaining after the solid cells and clotting factors have been removed.

serum electrolytes (e-lek'tro-litz)—the four principal cations and anions in the serum—sodium, chloride, potassium, and carbon dioxide.

sinus rhythm (si'nus)—the rate and rhythm of the heartbeat.

Skene's gland (skenz)—a gland in the female genitalia.

subcutaneous (sub-ku-ta'ne-us)—under the skin.

supine (su-pin')—lying on one's back.

suppurative (sup'u-ra-tiv)—forming pus.

suture (su'tur)—a surgical stitch—the thread-like material used to sew in surgery.

systolic (sis-tol'ik)—the higher number of the blood pressure.

T

thorax (tho'raks)—the bony rib cage that encloses the heart and lungs.

thrill—a visible or palpable motion in the chest wall corresponding to a heartbeat.

tissue (tish'u)—an aggregation of cells making up part of an organ.

tonsillectomy and adenoidectomy (T and A) (ton-si-lek'to-me) (ad-e-noi-dek'to-me)—removal of both the tonsil and adenoid glands.

trachea (tra'ke-ah)—wind pipe. (See Plates, I, VI, Appendix.)

transversalis fascia (trans-ver-sa'lis) (fash'yah)—thick fibrous tissue layer deep in abdominal wall.

transversus muscle (trans-ver'sus)—a deeper muscle of the abdominal wall.

tuberculosis (tu-ber-ku-lo'sis)—specific infectious disease, usually of the lungs.

U

umbilicus (um-bi-li'kus)—navel, belly button.

ureteral (u-re'ter-al)—referring to the ureter, the passageway or tube that leads urine from the kidney to the bladder.

urethra (u-re'thrah)—the portion of the urinary tract through which the urine flows from the bladder to outside the body. (See Plates IX, XII, Appendix.)

urinary (u'ri-ner-e)—relating to the kidneys, bladder.

uterus (u'ter-us)—the womb. (See Plate X, Appendix.)

V

varicella (var-i-sel'ah)—chicken pox.

vascularity (vas-ku-lar'i-te)—the degree or relative amount of blood vessels in an organ area.

vasculature (vas'ku-la-tur)—a composite of blood vessels.

W

white blood cell (WBC)—the solid matter in blood tissue is comprised, for the most part, of white and red blood cells. The white blood cells help fight infection.

WNL—within normal limits

Student: _____

Metropolitan Medical Center

HISTORY AND PHYSICAL EXAM

name   hospital no.

address   date of birth

                                                                              occupation

date   race

physician   room no.

Student: _____

Metropolitan Medical Center

X-RAY REPORT

name   **hospital no.**

age   **x-ray no.**

sex   **room no.**

physician   **date**

Student: _____

Metropolitan Medical Center

OPERATIVE RECORD

                    name   hospital no.

preoperative diagnosis   **room no.**

                                                       date

postoperative diagnosis

                                               first assistant
                                                 instrument
                      surgeon   **nurse**
second assistant   **sponge count**

circulating nurse

operation title or description

45

Student: _____

Metropolitan Medical Center

PATHOLOGY REPORT

name   hospital no.

tissue   room no.

date received   pathology
                                                             report no.

date reported

Student: _____

Metropolitan Medical Center

DISCHARGE SUMMARY

name　　　　　　　　　　　　　　　　　　　　　　**hospital no.**

admitted　　　　　　　　　　　　　　　　　　　　　**room no.**

discharged　　　　　　　　　　　　　　　　　　　　**age**

diagnosis

surgery

complications

special procedures

consultations

CASE B

Student: _____

name Bruce Babbs

address 720 Bellaire Court
El Cajon, CA 92020-1808

situation This 45-year-old male was found unconscious in the men's room at work and taken to the hospital in an ambulance. He was examined and a diagnosis of diabetic coma was made. He was seen in consultation by a specialist. X-ray tests were performed. He responded to treatment and was discharged.

In cases involving diabetes, an endocrinologist may be consulted. Endocrinology is a subspecialty of internal medicine and it deals with the disorders of the ductless glands. Special conditions of sterility, menopause, and disease of the adrenal and thyroid glands are treated by an endocrinologist.

Plate IX in the Appendix is related to this case.

sequence of reports

B-1
History and Physical Exam
Completed _____

B-2
Consultant's Report
Completed _____

B-3
X-ray Report
Completed _____

B-4
Discharge Summary
Completed _____

Note: Enter the date of completion for each report. When you have finished all the reports, tear this sheet out and give to your instructor along with the completed transcripts.

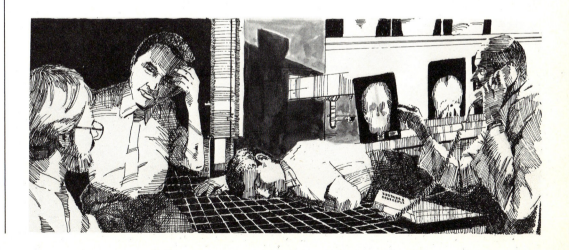

51

DEFINITIONS OF WORDS, PHRASES, AND ABBREVIATIONS

A

acetone (as'e-ton)—a chemical which has a sharp but fruity odor.
afebrile (a-feb'ril)—without fever.
Ampicillin (am-pi-si'lin)—trade name for a specific antibiotic.
anal (a'nal)—pertaining to the anus or external opening leading to the rectum.
antibiotic (an-te-bi-ot'ik)—a drug used to combat infection.

B

bacteriuria (bak-te-re-u're-ah)—bacteria in the urine.
benign (be-nin')—having no evidence of malignancy.
bilateral (bi-lat'er-al)—both sides of the body, or both organs of a system where there is one on each side of the body, such as kidneys, eyes, lungs.
boggy—being soft and compressible.
broad spectrum—referring to an antibiotic which is effective against a wide variety (or broad spectrum) of bacteria.

C

carotid (kah-rot'id)—the large artery on either side of the neck.
catheter (kath'e-ter)—a hollow tube constructed to pass into a body cavity, commonly into the urinary bladder to drain urine.
catheterization (kath-e-ter-i-za'shun)—the act of placing a catheter into the patient.
cholecystectomy (ko-le-sis-tek'to-me)—the operation in which the gallbladder is removed.
colony count—denotes the number of bacteria present in a given volume.
coma (ko'mah)—a state of unconsciousness.
comatose (ko-mah-tos')—being in a state of coma.
consolidation (kon-sol-e-da'shun)—when used in reference to the lungs, indicates a condition of abnormal solidity to the tissue with lack of normal air cells or spaces.

D

diabetes mellitus (di-ah-bet'tez) (mel'i-tus)—a metabolic disorder in which the oxidation of carbohydrates is reduced.
diabetic (di-ah-bet'ik)—pertaining to diabetes.
diarrhea (di-ah-re'ah)—abnormal frequency and softness of fecal elimination.
distention (dis-ten'shun)—the state of being enlarged or engorged.
dorsal (dor'sal)—on the back of, referring to the back.

E

endocrinology (en-do-krin-ol'o-je)—the study of the endocrine glands (the internally secreting glands of the body).
Escherichia coli (E. coli)—a genus of bacteria found in the alimentary canal.
excretion (eks-kre'shun)—the act or function of excreting which is to discharge or throw off waste material.

F

febrile (feb'ril)—having a fever.
femoral (fem'or-al)—referring to the femur (thigh bone).
flatulence (flat'u-lens)—excessive gas in the stomach or intestines.
Foley catheter (kath'e-ter)—a type of catheter which can be left in the bladder to drain urine, devised by Dr. Foley.

G

gait disturbances—refers to an abnormal walk or stagger.
glycosuria (gli-ko-su're-ah)—sugar in the urine.
guaiac (gwi'ak)—a test performed on stool specimens to check for the presence of blood.

H

hyperglycemia (hi-per-gli-se'me-ah)—having too much sugar in the blood.
hyperpneic (hi-perp'ne-ik)—state of breathing characterized by rapid respiration.
hypesthesia (hi-pes-the'ze-ah)—a condition of decreased sensation to touch or pinprick of the skin.
hypoactive (hi-po-ak'tiv)—having diminished or lessened activity or function.
hypotensive (hi-po-ten'siv)—having an abnormally low blood pressure.

I

icterus (ik'ter-us)—a yellow color—jaundice.
ingestion (in-jes'chun)—the act of taking food or liquid into the stomach.
insulin (in'su-lin)—a hormone (normally produced by the pancreas) which is deficient in diabetes.
intercostal (in-ter-kos'tal)—between the ribs.
intravenous (in-trah-ve'nus)—injected directly into a vein.
intravenous pyelogram (IVP) (in-trah-ve'nus) (pi'el-o-gram)—excretory urography.

K

Keflex (ke'fleks)—a specific type of broad spectrum antibiotic.
ketoacidosis (ke-to-as-e-do'sis)—a specific state of chemical imbalance seen in uncontrolled diabetes.

M

macula (mak'u-lah)—a specific anatomic spot on the retina which is the most light sensitive.
malleolus (mal-e'o-lus)—the bony prominence on the inside and outside of each ankle.
melena (mel-e'na)—black or tarry stools.
midclavicular (mid-klah-vik'u-lar)—an imaginary anatomical reference line drawn vertically down the body from the midpoint of the clavicle or collarbone.

N

NPH—isophane insulin suspension.

O

obtunded (ob-tund′ed)—in a stupor.
ocular (ok′u-lar)—pertaining to the eye.
orthopnea (or-thop′ne-ah)—difficulty in breathing while lying flat.

P

paresthesias (par-es-the′ze-as)—a "pins and needles" feeling in the skin.
pedal (ped′al)—pertaining to the foot.
phallus (fal′us)—the male sex organ (penis).
PMI—point of maximum impulse
popliteal (pop-lit-e′al)—an anatomical area referring to the back of the knee.
prostate (pros′tat)—an accessory reproductive organ in the male.
prostatitis (pros-tah-ti′tis)—an inflammation of the prostate gland.
psoas (so′as)—a muscle in the back wall of the abdomen.
punctate (punk′tat)—pinpoint.

pyelocalyceal (pi-el-o-kal-e-se′al)—referring to the internal collecting system of the kidney.
pyuria (pi-u′re-ah)—pus in the urine.

R

rales (rahls)—soft, bubbly, abnormal breathing sounds heard on listening to the lungs.
rectally (rek′tal-le)—pertaining to the rectum.
retinal (ret′i-nel)—the retina or inner lining of the fundus of the eye.
retinopathy (ret-i-nop′ah-the)—a disease in the retina.
rhonchi (rong′ki)—abnormal harsh breathing sounds heard on listening to the lungs with a stethoscope.
Ringer's lactate (lak′tat)—a type of intravenous fluid given to restore body chemical balance.

S

sequelae (se-kwe′li)—after effects or complications.
sinus (si′nus)—referring to the "sinal node" or natural pacemaker of the heart.
sinus tachycardia (tak-e-kar′de-ah)—a rapid heart rate, but produced in a regular rhythm by the natural pacemaker or sinal node of the heart.

sphincter (sfingk′ter)—a circular muscle surrounding an orifice capable of opening and closing that orifice.

T

tachycardia (tak-e-kar′de-ah)—a rapid heart rate.
tendon (ten′dun)—the dense connective tissue band joining muscle to bone.
testes (tes′tes)—the plural of testis or testicle.
trauma (traw′mah)—injury.
trophic (trof′ik)—resulting from interruption of blood or nerve supply.

U

ureter (u′re-ter)—the passageway or tube that leads urine from the kidney to the bladder. (See Plate IX, Appendix.)

V

venous (ve′nus)—pertaining to the noun vein.
vertigo (ver′te-go)—dizziness.
void—describes the act of urination.

W

WBC—white blood count

Student: _____

Metropolitan Medical Center

HISTORY AND PHYSICAL EXAM

name   hospital no.

address   date of birth

                                        occupation

date   race

physician   room no.

Student: _____

Metropolitan Medical Center

CONSULTANT'S REPORT

to   hospital no.

from   room no.

re   date

reason for consultation

Student: _____

Metropolitan Medical Center

X-RAY REPORT

name	**hospital no.**
age	**x-ray no.**
sex	**room no.**
physician	**date**

Student: _____

Metropolitan Medical Center

DISCHARGE SUMMARY

name											hospital no.

admitted										room no.

discharged										age

diagnosis

surgery

complications

special
procedures

consultations

CASE C

Student: _____

name Clarence Carroll

address 468 Burwick
La Jolla, CA 92037-2007

situation This 62-year-old man was first noticed by his wife kneeling on the floor in his workshop clutching his chest and struggling for breath. He was taken to the hospital by ambulance. Initial evaluation was not conclusive. He was seen in consultation by a pulmonary disease specialist and with the aid of special tests, a diagnosis of a blood clot in the lung (pulmonary embolism) was made. Pulmonary diseases are disorders of the lungs and respiratory system. Treatment was successful and he was discharged 13 days later.

Plates I and II in the Appendix are related to this case.

sequence of reports

C-1
History and Physical Exam
Completed _____

C-2
X-ray Report
Completed _____

C-3
X-ray Report (Lung Scan)
Completed _____

C-4
Consultant's Report
Completed _____

C-5
Discharge Summary
Completed _____

Note: Enter the date of completion for each report. When you have finished all the reports, tear this sheet out and give to your instructor along with the completed transcripts.

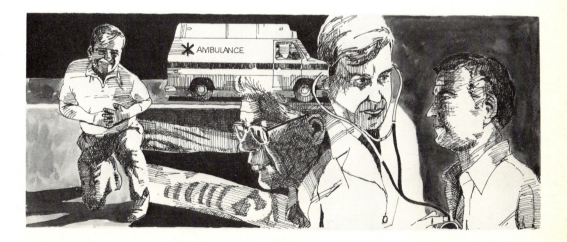

Transcribe Cassette Quiz No. 1 on the form found on page 77 before starting to work on Case D.

DEFINITIONS OF WORDS, PHRASES, AND ABBREVIATIONS

A

analgesic (an-al-je'zik)—pain killing drug.
angina (an'jin-ah)—severe pain in the chest, produced by heart disease.
anterior (an-te're-or)—in the front, or on the front side.
anteroposterior (AP)—X-ray beam passes from front to back.
anticoagulant (an-te-ko-ag'u-lant)—a medicine to prevent clotting of the blood.
appendectomy (ap-en-dek'to-me)—removal of the appendix.
arterial blood gases (ar-te're-al)—a test to measure the amount of dissolved oxygen and carbon dioxide in the blood.

B

basal (ba'sal)—the lowermost or bottom part of an organ.
bundle branch block—referring to a defect of conduction of a nerve impulse to the heart muscle.

C

cardiogram (kar'de-o-gram)—shortened form for electrocardiogram.
cardiothoracic (kar-de-o-tho-ras'ik)—the composite of heart and lungs.
cardiothoracic ratio—a measurement of the heart size as seen on X-ray film as compared to the size of the chest cavity.
closed reduction—describes the setting of a fractured bone into proper alignment (reduction) without resort to surgery (closed).
codeine (ko'den)—a frequently used pain killer.
colon (ko'lon)—general term for the large bowel.
colonic (ko-lon'ik)—referring to the colon.
consolidative (kon-sol-e-da'tiv)—having a tendency to consolidate or become solid and firm.
contusion (kon-tu'zhun)—a bruise.
costophrenic (kos-to-fren'ik)—adjective describing an area at the junction of rib (costo) and diaphragm (phrenic).
Coumadin (koo'mah-din)—trade name for a blood-thinning medicine designed to prevent clotting, an anticoagulant.
crepitant (krep'i-tant)—crackling.
crepitant rales (krep'i-tant rahls)—abnormal crackling sounds heard on auscultation of the chest.
culture (kul'tur)—denotes the placing of a specimen of body fluid or tissue in a certain environment so that any organisms present in that specimen will proliferate and thus can be identifiable.
cutaneous (ku-ta'ne-us)—pertaining to the skin.
cyanosis (si-ah-no'sis)—having a bluish color as when tissue is deprived of oxygen.

D

diaphragmatic (di-ah-frag-mat'ik)—pertaining to the diaphragm.
differential (dif-er-en'shal)—referring to the differential count of the various types of white blood cells noted in a specimen of blood.

E

effusion (ef-u'zhun)—escape of fluid into a body cavity.
EKG (electrocardiogram)—the graphic record obtained with the electrocardiograph of the heart's current action.
embolization (em-bo-li-za'shun)—the act of forming an embolus or blood clot.
embolus (em'bo-lus) or **embolism** (em'bo-lizm)—a blood clot.
epigastric (ep-e-gas'trik)—the middle upper part of the abdomen just below the rib cage.
erythema (er-e-the'mah)—redness of the skin, inflammation.
ethanol (eth'ah-nol)—the alcohol such as is in whiskey, beer, and wine.
excursion (eks-kur'shun)—up-and-down or side-to-side movement.
extraocular (eks-tra-ok'u-lar)—outside of the eye.

F

fossa (fos'ah); plural, **fossae** (fos'a)—a hole or indentation.
fossa ovalis (fos'ah) (o-val'-is)—an oval fossa or hole, such as where an artery, nerve, or vein penetrates deep into the tissue or bone.
friction rub—an abnormal sound heard on auscultation of the chest caused by two rough surfaces rubbing against each other.

H

hemoptysis (he-mop'tis-is)—coughing of blood.
Heparin (hep'ah-rin)—trade name for an anticoagulant drug given by injection.
hepatomegaly (hep-ah-to-meh'-ga-le)—enlargement of the liver.
herniorrhaphy (her-ne-or'ah-fe)—the name for a hernia operation or hernia repair.
hyperpnea (hi-perp'-ne-ah)—a state of breathing characterized by rapid respiration.

I

I.C.U.—intensive care unit
induration (in-du-ra'shun)—hardness.
infarct (in'farkt) or **infarction** (in-fark'shun)—describes death of tissue resulting from the sudden stoppage or interference with circulation of blood to that tissue.
infiltrate (in'fil-trat)—a collection of dense material.
inguinal (ing'gwi-nal)—pertaining to the groin area.
ischemia (is-ke'me-ah)—deficiency in blood, a compromise in the blood supply to an organ.
isotope (i'so-top)—a radioactive tracer substance injected into the body.

J

jugular (jug'u-lar)—the large vein in the neck.

L

lateral (lat′er-al)—referring to the side of an organ or body part.

M

mass (mas)—a general term for an abnormal solid structure of any size frequently representing a tumor or growth.

myocardial (mi-o-kar′de-al)—referring to the heart muscle.

myocardium (mi-o-kar′de-um)—the heart muscle.

O

oropharynx (o-ro-far′inks)—the composite anatomical term for mouth (oro) and throat (pharynx).

P

pathogen (path′o-jen)—an organism or bacterium capable of causing disease.

pCO2—partial pressure of carbon dioxide.

penicillin (pen-e-sil′in)—a commonly used antibiotic.

perfusion (per-fu′zhun)—the passage of fluid material through an organ.

pleura (ploor′ah)—the internal lining of the thorax (rib cage) and lung.

pleural (ploor′al)—referring to the pleura.

pleurisy (ploor′i-se)—inflammation of the pleura.

pleuritic (ploor-it′ik)—referring to the pleura.

pneumonic (nu-mon′ik)—referring to the lung or lungs.

pneumonitis (nu-mo-ni′tis)—pneumonia or inflammation of the lung.

pO2—partial pressure of oxygen.

polydipsia (pol-e-dip′se-ah)—excessive thirst.

polyp (pol′ip)—a finger-like fleshy growth.

polyphagia (pol-e-fa′je-ah)—excessive hunger.

polyuria (pol-e-u′re-ah)—excessive urination or larger than normal amounts of urine.

posterior (pos-te′re-or)—behind or on the back side.

posteroanterior (PA)—X-ray beam passes from back to front.

prothrombin (pro-throm′bin)—a constituent of the blood necessary for clotting.

prothrombin time—a laboratory test measuring the time it takes prothrombin to act in the formation of a clot.

pulmonic (pul-mon′ik)—referring to the lung.

R

Romberg—a specific abnormal nerve reflex named after Dr. Romberg.

right bundle branch block—referring to a defect of conduction of a nerve impulse to the heart muscle.

rule out—indicates the necessity to exclude a certain diagnostic possibility.

S

scan—a diagnostic procedure whereby an organ's function or capacity is determined by measuring the amount of an administrated radioactive tracer substance it picks up and contains.

sigmoid (sig′moid)—the lowest part of the large bowel nearest the rectum.

sigmoidoscope (sig-moid-o-skop′)—an instrument which can be introduced into the rectum to examine the sigmoid.

sigmoidoscopic (sig-moid-os-kop′-ik)—an examination of the sigmoid by a sigmoidoscope.

sputum (spu′tum)—the thick material produced by a cough.

sulcus (sul′kus); plural, **sulci** (sul′-si)—a trough or hollow.

T

thrombophlebitis (throm-bo-fle-bi′-tis)—an inflammation of and clotting of blood in a vein.

thyroid (thi′roid)—a gland of internal secretion located in the neck overlying the windpipe (trachea).

tibia (tib′e-ah)—the large bone in the leg from the knee to the ankle. (See Plate IV, Appendix.)

two plus enlarged—a system of grading the degree of a particular phenomenon, such as enlargement.

V

varicocele (var′e-ko-sel)—varicose veins in the scrotum.

varicose (var′e-kos)—dilated and tortuous (varicose veins).

varicosities (var-e-kos′i-tez)—referring to varicose veins.

ventricle (ven′tre-kl)—a large heart chamber. (See Plate VIII, Appendix.)

ventricular (ven-trik′u-lar)—referring to the ventricle.

vital signs—the broadest signs of the patient's general condition (the pulse, temperature, respiration, and blood pressure).

Student: _____

Metropolitan Medical Center

HISTORY AND PHYSICAL EXAM

name   hospital no.

address   date of birth

                                                            occupation

date   race

physician   room no.

Student: _____

Metropolitan Medical Center

X-RAY REPORT

name   hospital no.

age   x-ray no.

sex   room no.

physician   date

Student: _____

Metropolitan Medical Center

X-RAY REPORT

name   hospital no.

age   x-ray no.

sex   room no.

physician   date

Student: _____

Metropolitan Medical Center

CONSULTANT'S REPORT

to   hospital no.

from   room no.

re   date

reason for consultation

Student: _____

Metropolitan Medical Center

DISCHARGE SUMMARY

name   hospital no.

admitted   room no.

discharged   age

diagnosis

surgery

complications

special procedures

consultations

Cassette Quiz No. 1   Student: _____

Metropolitan Medical Center
HISTORY AND PHYSICAL EXAM

name   hospital no.

address   date of birth

                                         occupation

date   race

physician   room no.

CASE D

Student: _____

name Dorothy Deland

address 2401 Ginger Way
Oceanside, CA 92056-1075

situation This 25-year-old-woman was admitted to the hospital because of severe abdominal pain and vaginal bleeding. After an initial evaluation and X-ray study, she was taken to surgery where examination and surgical exploration revealed an ectopic pregnancy which was removed. The pathology report confirmed the diagnosis. She convalesced well and was discharged home one week after admission.

An ectopic pregnancy occurs when a fertilized ovum implants itself in one of the fallopian tubes rather than in the uterus, as would be the case in a normal pregnancy. As the fetus grows, the tube ruptures and presents the danger of hemorrhage.

Study and treatment of the female reproductive system is handled by a specialist in gynecology and obstetrics. Obstetrics is concerned with pregnancy, prenatal care, childbirth, and postpartum care. Gynecology is concerned with disorders of the female reproductive organs.

Refer to Plate X in the Appendix for additional information pertaining to this case.

sequence of reports

D-1
History and Physical Exam
Completed _____

D-2
X-ray Report
Completed _____

D-3
Operative Record
Completed _____

D-4
Pathology Report
Completed _____

D-5
Discharge Summary
Completed _____

Note: Enter the date of completion for each report. When you have finished all the reports, tear this sheet out and give to your instructor along with the completed transcripts.

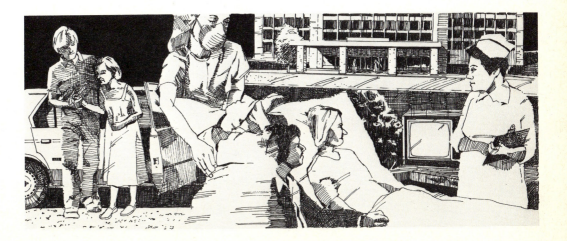

Complete the written quiz on page 95 before submitting your work on this case. Follow the directions of your instructor for checking your answers.

DEFINITIONS OF WORDS, PHRASES, AND ABBREVIATIONS

A

adnexa—(ad-nek'sah)—parts accessory to the main organ.
air-fluid levels—a finding on an abdominal X-ray where fluid settles in the bowel and an air shadow is seen above it.
ambulate (am'bu-lat)—to walk, to be up and about.
anorexic (an-o-rek'sik)—having anorexia.
anteverted (an-te-vert'ed)—flexed or tilted forward.
apical (ap'e-kal)—the apex or point of a roughly triangular structure.
areola (ah-re'o-lah); plural, **areolae** (a-re'o-la)—the pigmented area around the nipples.
arthralgia (ar-thral'je-ah)—pain in the bones or joints.
arthritis (ar-thri'tis)—inflammation of a bone joint.
auditory (aw'de-tor-re)—relating to the sense of hearing.
avascular (a-vas'ku-lar)—without blood or a blood supply.
axilla (ak-sil'ah); plural, **axillae** (ak-sil'a)—the armpit.

B

bimanual (bi-man'u-al)—using both hands to examine.

C

cannula (kan'u-lah)—a hollow surgical instrument used to drain or inspect an organ.
carbon dioxide (kar'bon) (di-ok'sid)—the inert gas frequently used to distend a body cavity and facilitate observation.
cervical canal—the passage within the cervix.
chorionic (ko-re-on'ik)—referring to the fetal membrane (chorion), an early state of development in a fertilized egg.
culdocentesis (kul-do-sen-te'sis)—inspection of the pelvic organs by an instrument introduced through the vaginal wall.
curettage (ku-re-tahzh')—the act of scraping the interior of a hollow organ to remove tissue from within.
cystitis (sis-ti'tis)—inflammation of the urinary bladder.

D

D and C (dilation and curettage)—dilation of the cervix and curettage of the lining of the uterus.
decompensation (de-kom-pen-sa'shun)—a state of fatigue or inefficiency.
Dexon (dek'son)—a specific type of absorbable suture.
dilation (di-la'shun)—the act of dilating or enlarging a certain organ by stretching.
dilate (di'lat)—to stretch or enlarge.
dissection (di-sek'shun)—inspection by cutting apart or separating tissues.
diverticulitis (di-ver-tik-u-li'tis)—inflammation of a diverticulum.
diverticulum (di-ver-tik'u-lum)—a weakened area (or blow out) in the wall of a hollow structure.
dorsal lithotomy position (lith-ot'o-me)—a position used for many vaginal and bladder examinations and procedures.
dysmenorrhea (dis-men-o-re'ah)—a painful menstrual period.
dysphagia (dis-fa'je-ah)—difficulty swallowing.

E

ectopic (ek-top'ik)—an organ or structure which is in a position other than its normal anatomical place.
ectopic gestation (jes-ta'shun)—a pregnancy occurring in a cavity other than the uterus or womb.
ectopic pregnancy—tubal pregnancy.
emesis (em'e-sis)—vomiting.
engorgement (en-gorj'ment)—excessive fullness of an organ.
exquisite (eks'kwi-zit)—describes pain or tenderness of the highest and most intense degree.

F

fallopian tube (fah-lo'pe-an)—the tube leading from the ovary to the uterus conducting the egg to the womb where it will develop. (See Plate X, Appendix.)
fimbria (fim'bre-ah)—the delicate finger-like projections at the end of the fallopian tube nearest the ovary.

G

gestation (jes-ta'shun)—pregnancy.
grade system—used to delineate the relative size of an organ or intensity of a sound, Grade 0 being the lowest and Grade VI usually the highest.
gynecologist (gin-e-kol'o-jist)—a physician who specializes in the treatment of disease of the female reproductive and genital systems.

H

hematochezia (hem-ah-to-ke'ze-ah)—passage of fresh blood in the stool.
hemorrhagic (hem-o-raj'ik)—bloody or containing blood.
hyperpigmented (hi-per-pig'mented)—having more than normal pigment, a dark coloration.
hypertension (hi-per-ten'shun)—abnormally high blood pressure.
hypotension (hi-po-ten'shun)—low blood pressure.

I

ileus formation (il'e-us)—obstruction of the bowel.
insufflated (in'suf-fla-ted)—introducing or passing gas into a hollow cavity to distend it.
intraperitoneal (in-trah-per-e-to-ne'al)—occurring within the peritoneal cavity.
isthmus (isth'mus)—denoting the narrowed area of an organ.

L

laparoscope (lap'ah-ro-skop)—a hollow instrument used to insert into the abdomen to inspect the organs.

laparoscopy (lap-ah-ros'ko-pe)—a procedure whereby the interior of the abdomen is inspected by an instrument introduced through the abdomen wall.

laparotomy (lap-ah-rot'o-me)—an operation to explore the abdominal contents.

ligament (lig'ah-ment)—a dense (usually band-like) fibrous tissue structure connecting muscle to muscle or one organ to another.

liter (le'ter)—a metric measurement of approximately one quart.

lithotomy (lith-ot'o-me)—an operation to remove a stone.

lumbar (lum'bar)—referring to the low back.

lumen (lu'men)—the interior space of a tube-like structure.

lymph (limf)—a clear, sometimes faintly milky, fluid that is collected from the tissues in the body and flows through lymphatic channels to join the blood in veins.

lymphadenopathy (lim-fad-e-nop'ah-the)—enlargement or inflammation of the lymph glands.

lymph gland—numerous and various small glands throughout the body that act as filters to the lymph fluid.

M

meatus (me-a'tus)—the opening of an organ.

menorrhagia (men-or-ra'je-ah)—excessive bleeding during a menstrual period.

mesosalpinx (mes-o-sal'pinks)—the connective tissue bands or tethers holding the fallopian tube (salpinx) in place.

metrorrhagia (met-ro-ra'je-ah)—irregular bleeding from the uterus (through the vagina) in between menstrual periods.

millimeter (mil'e-me-ter)—a metric measurement of length.

mitral (mi'tral)—one of the heart valves (the mitral valve).

mitral insufficiency—a heart disease or defect caused by an abnormality (insufficiency) of the mitral valve in the heart.

mucosa (mu-ko'sah)—the thin membrane lining the interior of a hollow organ.

N

nodes (nodz)—refers to lymph nodes or lymph glands.

normal saline (sa'len)—a salt water solution, the concentration of which is physiological, and is compatible with the tissue of the body.

O

ophthalmoscopic (of-thal-mo-skop'-ik)—an examination by the ophthalmoscope or instrument one uses to examine the eye.

oral contraceptive (kon-trah-sep'tiv)—birth control pills.

outpatient (out'pa-shent)—a patient who is seen and followed outside of the hospital, such as a clinic or a doctor's office.

ovary (o'vah-re)—the female reproductive organ which produces the egg. (See Plate X, Appendix.)

P

palpable (pal'pah-bl)—perceptible by touch.

palpitations (pal-pi-ta'shunz)—unusually rapid action of the heart which is felt by the patient.

pathological (path-o-loj'e-kal)—abnormal or diseased.

pathology (pah-thol'o-je)—the study of disease and diseased tissue.

pelvic (pel'vik)—pertaining to the pelvis.

pelvis (pel'vis)—the lowermost part of the trunk of the body above the legs.

peritoneal cavity (per-i-to-ne'al)—the interior of the abdomen containing all of the abdominal organs.

peritonitis (per-i-to-ni'tis)—inflammation of the peritoneum.

Pfannenstiel incision (pfahn'en-stel)—a curved, lower abdominal incision named after Johann Pfannenstiel, a German gynecologist.

prophylactic (pro-fi-lak'tik)—something taken or done as a preventative measure to disease.

R

rectus muscles (rek'tus)—the midline abdominal muscles.

reflex (re'fleks); plural, **reflexes** (re'fleks-is)—response to stimuli.

reprepped and redraped—act of repositioning the patient, prepping (cleaning), and draping the surgical area.

resect (re-sekt')—to surgically remove.

retracting (re-trak'ting)—the act of drawing back the edges of a wound or incision.

rheumatic (ru-mat'ik)—relating to rheumatism.

rheumatic heart disease—heart disease acquired in the course of rheumatic fever.

rheumatism (ru'mah-tizm)—various symptoms of the bones and joints.

rheumatoid (ru'mah-toid)—referring to a rheumatic condition.

round ligament—a specific ligament in the female pelvis helping to suspend the uterus.

rupture (rup'chur)—a break in any organ.

S

saline (sa'len)—a salt water solution.

salpingectomy (sal-pin-jek'to-me)—removal of a fallopian tube.

scoliosis (sko-le-o'sis)—an abnormal curvature or rotation of the spine.

shocky (sho'ke)—being in a state of shock.

sibling (sib'ling)—a brother or sister.

spotty (spot'e)—used to describe vaginal bleeding as scant and intermittent.

subcuticular (sub-ku-tik'u-lar)—the part of the skin just below the outer layer.

subumbilical (sub-um-bil'e-kal)—below (sub) the belly button (umbilicus).

symptoms (simp'tums)—denotes the specific complaints a patient offers regarding an illness.

T

tenaculum (te-nak'u-lum)—a surgical instrument used to grasp an organ.

tonsillitis (ton-si-li′tis)—inflammation of the tonsils.

tonsils (ton′silz)—small glands in the throat situated near the back of the tongue.

tubal (tu′bal)—referring to the fallopian tube.

tubal pregnancy—one occurring in the fallopian tube.

tubal stump—the blind end of the tube after the main part has been resected.

U

upright (up′rit)—in this sense referring to an X-ray of an area taken with the patient standing.

urethral (u-re′thral)—referring to the urethra.

uterine (u′ter-in)—referring to the uterus or womb.

V

vaginal (vaj′i-nal)—referring to the vagina or birth canal. (See Plate X, Appendix.)

villi (vil′e)—finger-like projections of microscopic size.

visual (vizh′u-al)—relating to the sense of sight.

Student: _____

Metropolitan Medical Center

HISTORY AND PHYSICAL EXAM

name   hospital no.

address   date of birth

                                             occupation

date   race

physician   room no.

Student: _____

Metropolitan Medical Center

X-RAY REPORT

name   hospital no.

age   x-ray no.

sex   room no.

physician   date

Student: _____

Metropolitan Medical Center

OPERATIVE RECORD

name   hospital no.

preoperative diagnosis   room no.

                                         date

postoperative diagnosis

                                       first assistant
                                       instrument
              surgeon   nurse
second assistant   sponge count

circulating nurse

operation title or
description

Student: _____

Metropolitan Medical Center

PATHOLOGY REPORT

name　　　　　　　　　　　　　　　　　　　　　　**hospital no.**

tissue　　　　　　　　　　　　　　　　　　　　　　**room no.**

date received　　　　　　　　　　　　　　　　　　**pathology report no.**

date reported

Student: _____

Metropolitan Medical Center

DISCHARGE SUMMARY

name	hospital no.

admitted	room no.

discharged	age

diagnosis

surgery

complications

special
procedures

consultations

Written Quiz No. 1

Name _____

Date _____

Score _____

SECTION I

Directions: In the Answers column write the appropriate word from the vocabulary list below that defines the statement.

anorexia	cutaneous	guaiac	saline
Babinski	cyanosis	hematemesis	scoliosis
carotid	ectopic	lesion	trachea
cecum	edema	pleura	vertigo
	embolus	renal	

                                                              Answers   **For Scoring**

1. Internal lining of the thorax .... _____ 1. _____
2. Vomiting of blood .... _____ 2. _____
3. Curvature of the spine .... _____ 3. _____
4. Lack of appetite .... _____ 4. _____
5. Bluish discoloration from lack of oxygen .... _____ 5. _____
6. A neurological test .... _____ 6. _____
7. A salt solution .... _____ 7. _____
8. Pertaining to the kidney .... _____ 8. _____
9. A large artery in the neck .... _____ 9. _____
10. Dizziness .... _____ 10. _____
11. Referring to the skin .... _____ 11. _____
12. The windpipe .... _____ 12. _____
13. Abnormal finding (a growth) .... _____ 13. _____
14. Swelling .... _____ 14. _____
15. A blood clot .... _____ 15. _____
16. First part of large bowel .... _____ 16. _____
17. Out of place .... _____ 17. _____
18. A test for blood in feces .... _____ 18. _____

SECTION II

Directions: For each organ listed on the right, match three words or phrases from the list on the left that pertain to that particular organ.

		Answers	For Scoring
consolidation		Abdomen	
epigastric	1. _____		1. ____
external oblique muscle	2. _____		2. ____
extraocular	3. _____		3. ____
gallop			
macula		Eye	
murmur			
peritoneum	4. _____		4. ____
rales	5. _____		5. ____
rhonchi	6. _____		6. ____
sclerae			
ventricle		Heart	
	7. _____		7. ____
	8. _____		8. ____
	9. _____		9. ____
		Lung	
	10. _____		10. ____
	11. _____		11. ____
	12. _____		12. ____

SECTION III

Directions: In the space provided write the meaning of each of these commonly used abbreviations or chemical symbols.

	Answers	For Scoring
1. DTR	_____	1. ____
2. EKG	_____	2. ____
3. E.R.	_____	3. ____
4. I.C.U.	_____	4. ____
5. K	_____	5. ____
6. PTA	_____	6. ____
7. WBC	_____	7. ____
8. WNL	_____	8. ____

CASE E

Student: _____

name
Elaine Erenburg

address
5682 Kelsey Street
Santee, CA 92071-1852

situation
This 16-year-old girl was seriously injured in an auto accident and rushed to the medical center. She was given initial life-saving treatment in the shock-trauma unit. Various X-ray studies were done to evaluate the extent of her injury and she was brought to surgery. Her convalescence was lengthy, but her recovery was good, and she was discharged several weeks after admission.

Sometimes several specialists are required to work together in treating a patient. Because of the multiple internal injuries sustained in the accident, the specialties of general surgery, urology, and thoracic surgery were involved. Urology deals with disorders of the genitourinary tract of males and the urinary tract of females. The thoracic surgeon deals with surgical treatment of the thorax (chest). In this situation, more than one surgeon performed operative procedures during the same surgical time.

Plates III, IV, and IX in the Appendix are related to this case.

sequence of reports

E-1
History and Physical Exam
Completed _____

E-2
X-ray Report
Completed _____

E-3
Operative Record
Completed _____

E-4
Discharge Summary
Completed _____

Note: Enter the date of completion for each report. When you have finished all the reports, tear this sheet out and give to your instructor along with the completed transcripts.

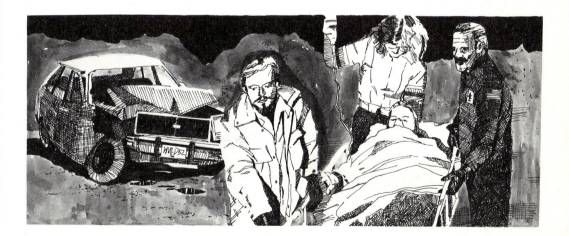

Transcribe Cassette Quiz No. 2 on the form found on Page 109 before starting work on Case F.

DEFINITIONS OF WORDS, PHRASES, AND ABBREVIATIONS

A

angulated (ang′gu-lat-ed)—broken off at an angle.
arteriosclerosis (ar-te-re-o-skle-ro′sis)—hardening of the arteries.
atelectasis (at-e-lek′tah-sis)—collapse of the lung.
auditory canal (aw′de-to-re)—the external ear canal.
axillary (ak′si-lar-e)—referring to the axillae or armpits.

B

bacteria (bak-te′re-ah)—germs, the small one celled organisms that cause infections.
basilar (bas′i-lar)—the base or lowermost part of an organ.
basilic (ba-sil′ik)—important or prominent

C

central venous pressure (ve′nus)—the blood pressure of the large internal veins in the body.
coagulase positive (ko-ag′u-las)—the characteristics of a bacterium, particularly staphylococcus.
comminuted (kom′in-ut-ed)—a fracture of bone which is broken into several different pieces.
contrast material—a liquid solution or dye which introduced into the body shows up sharply on X-ray.
coronary thrombosis (kor′o-na-re) (throm-bo′sis)—a blood clot in the main blood vessel nourishing the heart.
cranium (kra′ne-um)—the skull.
crepitus (krep′i-tus)—a crackling sound such as may be produced by the rubbing together of bone fragments.
crest—topmost point of a structure.
cross-match—finding or matching a unit of donor blood which resembles the recipient's blood as closely as possible.
cut down—describes an incision through the skin to isolate a large blood vessel so that a tube may be inserted.

cyanotic (si-ah-not′ik)—displaying cyanosis.
cystogram (sis′to-gram)—a special X-ray of the urinary bladder.
cystostomy (sis-tos′to-me)—the formation of an opening into the bladder.
cystotomy (sis-tot′o-me)—a surgical incision or opening made into the bladder.

D

diffuse (de-fus′)—spread out, not localized.
distal (dis′tal)—furthest part of a limb, bone, or organ away from the central point of the body.
doubly ligated (li′gat-ed)—to ligate twice.
duodenum (du-o-de′num)—that portion of the small bowel adjacent to the stomach. (See Plate II, Appendix.)

E

epicondylar fracture (ep-e-kon′dil-ar)—a fracture occurring through the epicondyle of a bone.
epicondyle (ep-e-kon′dil)—a bony prominence or knob which is situated just above the rounded joint surface of a bone.
extravasation (eks-trav-ah-sa′shun)—leakage from within the confines of an organ to surrounding areas.

F

febrile convulsions (feb′ril) (kon-vul′shunz)—seizures experienced during a high fever.
femur (fe′mur)—the thigh bone extending from the hip to the knee. (See Plate IV, Appendix.)
figure-of-eight sutures (su′turz)—sutures placed in the figure of the numeral eight.
fixation (fiks-a′shun)—denotes the bringing of fractured bones into proper alignment.
fixation pins (fiks-a′shun)—stablizing pins.
fracture (frak′tur)—a break or tear in a bone or other organ.

fundus (fun′dus)—that part of a hollow organ furthest removed from its opening.

G

gastric (gas′trik)—referring to the stomach.
gastric vessels (gas′trik) (ves′elz)—the blood vessels entering the stomach.

H

hemopneumothorax (he-mo-nu-mo-tho′raks)—a combination of pneumothorax and hemothorax.
hemothorax (he-mo-tho′raks)—a condition whereby blood escapes between the lung and the chest wall.
humerus (hu′mer-us)—the arm bone extending from the shoulder to the elbow. (See Plate IV, Appendix.)

I

ilium (il′e-um)—the side bone of the pelvis.
incision (in-sizh′un)—a cutting into of the body.
IPPB—intermittent positive pressure breathing

L

lacerated (las′er-at-ed)—torn or cut.
laceration (las-er-a′shun)—a wound made by tearing or cutting.
lavage (lah-vahzh′)—to wash or rinse.
lesser sac (sak)—a small pouch within the abdominal cavity.

M

medulla (me-dul′ah)—any soft marrow-like structure; here referring to the internal (marrow) cavity of the bone.
medullary (med′u-lar-e)—referring to a medulla.
midshaft—referring to the middle of the shaft or length of a bone.
monitoring (mon′i-tor-ing)—to monitor, to check or keep track of.

N

naris (na′ris); plural, **nares** (na′res)—the nostril(s).

noncontributory—used by the dictating physician in dismissing the historical review of an organ system as unimportant to the case at hand.

O

organism (or'gan-ism)—any individual animal or plant, here referring to a bacterium.
orthopedic (or-tho-pe'dik)—the correction of deformity.
orthopedic surgeon—the bone surgeon or specialist.
osteomyelitis (os-te-o-mi-e-li'tis)—an infection of bone.

P

palpated (pal'pat-ed)—the act of feeling with the hands.
pedicle (ped'e-kel)—in this concept the area of an organ where the major nutrient blood vessels enter.
Penrose drain—a thin piece of soft rubber tube of varying lengths left in a body cavity or space, and brought to the exterior to drain accumulating blood and fluid to the outside.
perforation (per-fo-ra'shun)—a tear or opening into.
peripheral (peh-rif'er-al)—referring to the periphery (away from or peripheral to the central axis or trunk of the body).
philtrum (fil'trum)—the groove in the middle of the upper lip.
pneumothorax (nu-mo-tho'raks)—a condition whereby air escapes between the lung and chest wall.
portable—able to be moved about freely.
porta hepatis (por'tah) (he-pat'is)—the area on the underside of the liver where the blood vessels enter and the bile duct exits.
proteus (pro'te-us)—a type of bacterium.
pubis (pu'bis)—the pubic bone.

R

rectus fascia (rek'tus) (fash'e-ah)—the tough connective tissue (fascia) covering the rectus muscles (the middle muscles of the abdomen).
retention sutures—very strong sutures through all the layers of an incision to give added strength to a surgical closure.
retroperitoneal (re-tro-per-i-to-ne'al)—behind the peritoneum.

S

sacroiliac joint (sa-kro-il'e-ak)—the point where the sacrum and the ilium bones meet.
sacrum (sa'krum)—the lowermost large back bone just above the tail bone.
semicomatose (sem-e-ko-mah-tos')—nearly unconscious.
sensitivity (sen-si-tiv'i-te)—applied to bacteria indicating they are susceptible to eradication by the administration of a certain antibiotic.
shock (shok)—a state of serious body malfunction where the blood pressure drops, the pulse rate rises.
shock trauma unit—special area in the hospital to deal with serious injuries (trauma) and patients in shock.
spleen (splen)—a blood-forming organ in the upper left hand corner of the abdomen. (See Plate II, Appendix.)
splenectomy (sple-nek'to-me)—removal of the spleen.
splenic (splen'ik)—referring to the spleen.
stabilizing pins—metal pins or rods hammered into bones so that traction devices may be applied.
stab incision—a short incision (or stab) through overlying skin and muscle.
staphylococcus aureus (staf-i-lo-kok'kus) (aw're-us)—a type of bacteria frequently abbreviated to staph.
sterile saline (ster'il) (sa'len)—saline (or salt water) prepared so as to be free of bacteria.
suprapubic (su-prah-pu'bik)—above the pubic bone.
symphysis (sim'fi-sis)—the line of junction between two bones.
symphysis pubis (sim'fi-sis) (pu'bis)—the line of junction between the two pubic bones of the pelvis.

T

thoracic (tho-ras'ik)—pertaining to the thorax or chest.
thrombosis (throm-bo'sis)—a blood clot forming within a blood vessel and blocking it off.
tracheostomy (tra-ke-os'to-me)—the placement of a tube into the windpipe (trachea) through an external incision.
traction (trak'shun)—the application of a pull or strain to a bone or muscle to bring it into alignment.
transfusion (trans-fu'zhun)—the transfer of blood from one subject to another.
transverse (trans-vers')—in a horizontal fashion, from side to side.
tympanic membranes (tim-pan'ik)—eardrum.
typed—the typing of blood.

U

urology (u-rol'o-je)—that specialty of medicine which deals with the genitourinary tract.

V

viral (vi'ral)—referring to or caused by a virus.

X

xiphoid (zif'oid)—the lowest part of the breast bone.

Student: _____

Metropolitan Medical Center

HISTORY AND PHYSICAL EXAM

name

address

date

physician

hospital no.

date of birth

occupation

race

room no.

Student: _____

Metropolitan Medical Center

X-RAY REPORT

name   hospital no.

age   x-ray no.

sex   room no.

physician   date

Student: _____

Metropolitan Medical Center

OPERATIVE RECORD

name

preoperative diagnosis

postoperative diagnosis

surgeon
second assistant

circulating nurse

operation title or
description

hospital no.

room no.

date

first assistant
instrument
nurse
sponge count

Student: _____

Metropolitan Medical Center

DISCHARGE SUMMARY

name   hospital no.

admitted   room no.

discharged   age

diagnosis

surgery

complications

special
procedures

consultations

Cassette Quiz No. 2   Student: _____

Metropolitan Medical Center
OPERATIVE RECORD

name

preoperative diagnosis

postoperative diagnosis

surgeon
second assistant

circulating nurse

operation title or
description

hospital no.

room no.

date

first assistant
instrument
nurse
sponge count

CASE F

Student: _____

name Frank Forch

address 2139 Stanton Road
San Diego, CA 92105-1614

situation This 7-year-old boy was admitted to the Ear, Nose, and Throat Department of the hospital for surgery because of repeated ear infections. His ears were drained and infected tissue was removed at surgery. This procedure is referred to as a tympanotomy. The pathology report indicated chronic infection without evidence of any malignancy. He did well after surgery and was discharged to further office follow-up.

The specialty involved with the structure, function, and disorders of the ear, nose, and throat is otorhinolaryngology. Children are often seen by a pediatrician, a doctor who specializes in the treatment of children and the diseases commonly associated with children.

Plates in the Appendix related to this case are Plates I, VII, and XI.

sequence of reports

F-1
History and Physical Exam
Completed _____

F-2
Operative Record
Completed _____

F-3
Pathology Report
Completed _____

F-4
Discharge Summary
Completed _____

Note: Enter the date of completion for each report. When you have finished all the reports, tear this sheet out and give to your instructor along with the completed transcripts.

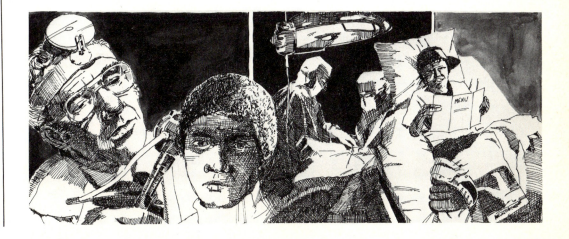

DEFINITIONS OF WORDS, PHRASES, AND ABBREVIATIONS

A

adenoidal (ad-e-noid'al)—referring to the adenoids.
adenoids (ad'e-noidz)—lymph glands in the back of the throat.
adhesions (ad-he'zhunz)—strands of scar tissue.
adrenalin (ad-ren'al-in)—brand name for a commonly used solution to constrict blood vessels.
anteriorly—(an-te're-or-le)—in front or on the front side.
anulus (an'u-lus)—a ring or ring-shaped structure.
asthma (az'mah)—a condition of difficult breathing characterized by gasping and wheezing.
aural (aw'ral)—relating to the ear.

B

bronchitis (brong-ki'tis)—an inflammation of the bronchus.
bronchus (brong'kus)—an air tube or passage within the lung leading eventually to the trachea or windpipe. (See Plate I, Appendix.)

C

chronic (kron'ik)—not acute, of long standing.
chronically (kron'-i-ka-le)—an adjective or adverb derived from chronic.
conductive hearing loss—hearing loss caused by a blockage or obstruction in the ear so that sound cannot pass (be conducted) within.
congestion (kon-jest'yun)—an accumulation of excessive fluid or blood in an organ.
Cortisporin (kor-te-spo'rin)—a brand name for a commonly used medication which helps prevent inflammation and promotes healing.
crypts (kriptz)—tiny pockets or indentations.
curette (ku-ret')—a surgical instrument used to scrape.

D

debridement (da-bred-maw')—the surgical exercise of removal of all unhealthy tissue from an area.
discharge (dis'-charj)—emission or drainage of fluid.

E

edematous (e-dem'ah-tus)—pertaining to or affected by edema.
enuresis (en-u-re'sis)—bed wetting.
epithelial (ep-e-the'le-al)—referring to the epithelium.
epithelium (ep-e-the'le-um)—a thin layer of cells normally present as a covering or lining of many organs.
eustachian tube (u-sta'ke-an)—a passage leading from the middle ear to the nasopharynx. Named after Bartolommeo Eustachio, an Italian anatomist.
excision (ek-sizh'un)—an act of cutting away or taking out.

F

flap—the piece of tissue loosened by a surgical incision.
friable (fri'ah-bl)—having the tendency to bleed easily.

G

Gelfoam (jel'fom)—a brand name for a spongy material which helps control bleeding.
granulation tissue (gran-u-la'shun) (tish'u)—raw fleshy tissue, commonly known as proud flesh.

H

hernia (her'ne-ah)—the protrusion of a loop or knuckle of an organ or tissue through an abnormal opening.
hydrocephalus (hi-dro-sef'ah-lus)—fluid on the brain. A condition where the entire head is of a markedly enlarged size.
hypertrophic (hi-per-trof'ik)—overgrown.
hypertrophy (hi-per'tro-fe)—a proliferation or overgrowth of any type of tissue.

I

infiltrated (in-fil-trat'-ed)—causing a substance to permeate or spread through a tissue.
intubate (in'tu-bat)—placing a tube into.

K

keratin (ker'ah-tin)—a very hard substance composed mainly of protein which is a principal component of the outer layer of skin, hair, and nails.

L

lymphoid (lim'foid)—referring to lymph gland tissue.

M

malignancy (mah-lig'nan-se)—cancer.
mastoid (mas'toid)—a specific part of the skull bone situated near the ear. (See Plate VII, Appendix.)
mastoidectomy (mas-toid-ek'to-me)—removal of the mastoid sinus.
mouth gag—a gauze or rubber piece placed in the mouth to isolate a particular part of the mouth.

N

nasopharynx (na-zo-far'inks)—the air passage leading from the nose to the throat.

P

palate (pal'at)—the partition separating nasal and oral cavities.
pes planus (pez) (pla'nus)—flat feet.
petechiae (pe-te'ke-i)—small red dots caused by leakage of blood from the tiniest of blood vessels called capillaries.
plasma cells (plaz'mah)—a type of blood cell.
poly (pol'e) polymorphonuclear leukocyte.
polypoid (pol'e-poid)—polyp-like in appearance.
promontory (prom'on-to-re)—a bony projection.
punch forcep (punch) (for'sep)—surgical grasping instrument used to punch out holes in tissue.

purulent (pu'roo-lent)—consisting of or containing pus.

R

retardation (re-tar-da'shun)—delayed development.
roseola (ro-ze-o'lah)—a viral infection causing a high fever and characteristic skin rash.

S

sedimentation rate (sed-i-men-ta'-shun)—a nonspecific blood test to check for the presence of inflammation.
soft palate (pal'at)—that portion of the roof of the mouth which is furthest toward the back of the throat.
squamous (skwa'mus)—a special type of cell typically seen in the outer layer of skin.
stroma (stro'mah)—the underlying supportive tissue.
symmetrical (si-met're-kal)—equality in size and form of parts.

T

torus tubarius (to'rus) (tu-ba're-us)—a ridge of tissue behind the eustachian tube.
transcanal (trans-ka-nal')—across the (ear) canal.
Tylenol (ti'le-nol)—brand name for a drug commonly used to relieve fever and pain.
tympano-mastoiditis (tim-pah-no-mas-toyd-i'tus)—inflammation of both the tympanic membrane (eardrum) and the mastoid sinus (an organ within the bone behind the ear).
tympanotomy (tim-pah-not'o-me)—an incision into the eardrum.

U

uvula (u'vu-lah)—the soft fleshy projection hanging down from the soft palate in the back of the oropharynx.

V

vascularized (vas'ku-la-rizd)—having an abundance of blood vessels.

X

Xylocaine (zi'lo-kan)—a brand name for a commonly used local anesthetic.

Student: _____

Metropolitan Medical Center

HISTORY AND PHYSICAL EXAM

name   hospital no.

address   date of birth

                                        occupation

date   race

physician   room no.

Student: _____

Metropolitan Medical Center

OPERATIVE RECORD

name   hospital no.

preoperative diagnosis   room no.

           date

postoperative diagnosis

           first assistant
           instrument
surgeon   nurse
second assistant   sponge count

circulating nurse

operation title or
description

Student: _____

Metropolitan Medical Center

PATHOLOGY REPORT

name															hospital no.

tissue															room no.

date received													pathology report no.

date reported

Student: _____

Metropolitan Medical Center

DISCHARGE SUMMARY

name   hospital no.

admitted   room no.

discharged   age

diagnosis

surgery

complications

special
procedures

consultations

CASE G

Student: _____

name Gary Goldstein

address 724 El Cerrito Place
Poway, CA 92064-2045

situation This 64-year-old patient was admitted to the hospital in urinary retention. His history was reviewed and an initial evaluation done. X-ray studies helped to make a diagnosis, and surgery was deemed necessary to relieve his urinary obstruction. The condition is called benign prostatic hypertrophy. The tissue removed was benign. His hospital course and convalescence were uneventful and he was discharged well.

Problems of the genitourinary tract are the specialty of urologists, and this condition was treated surgically by performing a transurethral resection of the prostate.

Plates IX and XII in the Appendix are related to this case.

sequence of reports

G-1
History and Physical Exam
Completed _____

G-2
X-ray Report
Completed _____

G-3
Operative Record
Completed _____

G-4
Pathology Report
Completed _____

G-5
Discharge Summary
Completed _____

Note: Enter the date of completion for each report. When you have finished all the reports, tear this sheet out and give to your instructor along with the completed transcripts.

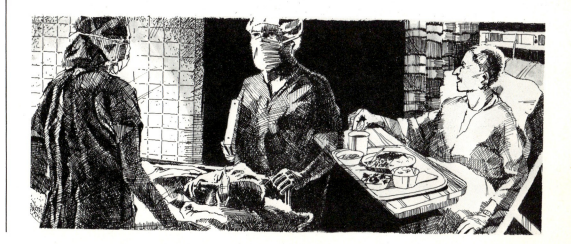

Complete the written quiz on page 137 before submitting your work for this case. Follow the directions of your instructor for checking your answers.

DEFINITIONS OF WORDS, PHRASES, AND ABBREVIATIONS

A

adenoma (ad-e-no'mah)—a benign fleshy growth of tissue.
ampulla (am-pul'ah)—flask-like, the dilated part of a hollow organ which takes on a flask-like shape.
anticholinergics (an-te-ko-lin-er'jiks)—medicine which controls stomach acidity and bowel overactivity.
apex (a'peks)—the point or tip of a roughly triangular structure.
arteriolar (ar-te-ri'o-lar)—referring to an arteriole.
arteriole (ar-te're-ol)—a small subdivision of an artery.
arteriosclerotic heart disease (ar-te-re-o-skle-rot'ik)—heart disease due to arteriosclerosis or hardening of the arteries.
atrophy (at'ro-fe)—shrinkage or diminution in size.
atypia (a-tip'e-ah)—abnormality, especially referring to abnormality in the cellular structure suggestive of cancer.

B

blood urea nitrogen (blud) (u-re'ah) (ni'tro-jen)—a blood test to measure the amount of urea nitrogen present in the body.
BPH—benign prostatic hypertrophy
bronchodilator (brong-ko-di'la-tor)—medication which expands the size of the bronchi or air passages of the lung, letting more air in.
bronchovascular (brong-ko-vas'ku-lar)—pertaining to both the bronchus and adjacent blood vessels.

C

calcification (kal-se-fi-ka'shun)—an object which has become calcified or turned to stone, or the state of having been calcified.
calyces (ka'li-sez)—the beginning of the collecting system in the kidney, small ducts that begin the passage of urine down the ureter to the bladder. (See Plate IX, Appendix.)
cardiac monitor (kar'de-ak)—a device to observe heart activity.
cellular (sel'u-lar)—pertaining to, or made up of cells.
cholelithiasis (ko-le-li-thi'ah-sis)—stones in the gallbladder.
cholesterol (ko-les'ter-ol)—a fat-like substance of the blood.
congestive (kon-jes'tiv)—having the characteristics of congestion.
cortisone (kor'te-son)—a drug to reduce swelling and inflammation.
cystoscope (sis'to-skop)—an instrument used to examine the urinary bladder and urethra.
cystoscopy (sis-tos'ko-pe)—an examination of the bladder carried out with a cystoscope.

D

degeneration (de-jen-er-a'shun)—deterioration.
degenerative (de-jen'er-a-tiv)—pertaining to the process of degeneration.
digitalis (dij-e-ta'lis)—a heart stimulating drug.
digitalized (dij'e-tal-izd)—the state of having been administered digitalis in effective doses.
duodenal (du-o-de'nal)—pertaining to the duodenum.

E

electrocardiographic (e-lek-tro-kar-de-o-gra'fik)—pertaining to an electrocardiogram.
electrocautery (e-lek-tro-kaw'ter-e)—a device used in surgery to staunch the flow of blood.
emphysema (em-fi-se'mah)—a disease of the lungs characterized by difficulty getting enough air.
excretory urography (eks'kre-to-re) (u-rog'rah-fe)—an intravenous pyelogram (an X-ray study of the kidney and ureter).
expiratory wheeze (eks-pir'a-to-re) (hwez)—a wheeze heard on expiration of air from the lung.
extrasystole (eks-trah-sis'to-le)—an extra beat of the heart, a skipped heartbeat.

F

feces (fe'sez)—the excrement discharged from the bowels.
fibromuscular (fi-bro-mus'ku-lar)—composed of both fibrous and muscular proportions.
fibrosis (fi-bro'-sis)—scar tissue.

G

genital (jen'e-tal)—pertaining to reproductive organs.
gland (gland)—a secreting organ, one that produces or secretes a special substance.
glandular (glan'du-lar)—made up of, or in the form of glands.
gram (gram)—a metric measure of weight.

H

hesitancy (hez'i-ten-se)—difficulty in starting the urinary stream.
histologic (his-to-loj'ik)—referring to histology.
histology (his-tol'o-je)—the study of tissue and cellular structure.
hydronephrosis (hi-dro-ne-fro'sis)—an abnormal collection of fluid within the kidney.
hyperaeration (hi-per-er-a'shun)—overly filled with air.
hyperemia (hi-per-e'me-ah)—engorgement with blood vessels.
hyperplasia (hi-per-pla'ze-ah)—an overgrowth of the tissue in an organ, or increase in organ size by an absolute increase in the number of cellular structures.
hyperresonant (hi-per-rez'o-nant)—exaggerated resonance.

I

inflammatory cells (in-flam'ah-to-re)—cells present in the process of inflammation.
interstitial (in-ter-stish'al)—pertaining to or situated within the interspaces or gaps of tissue.

intravenous pyelogram (in-trah-ve′nus) (pi′el-o-gram)—excretory urography.
irrigated (ir′i-gat-ed)—the state of being washed out or rinsed.

L

laminar (lam-i-nar)—layered or made up of different layers.
lobe (lob)—a part of an organ demarcated by an anatomical division.

M

metabolic (met-ah-bol′ik)—referring to metabolism.
metabolism (me-tab′o-lizm)—the energy process by which living tissue is maintained.

N

neoplasia (ne-o-pla′ze-ah)—new growth, usually refers to cancerous growth.
nitroglycerine (ni-tro-glis′er-in)—a medication which increases blood flow to the heart muscle.

O

occluded (ok-klud′ed)—the state of being closed tight.
orifice (or′i-fis); plural, **orifices** (or′i-fi-sez)—an opening into an organ or structure.

P

panendoscope (pan-en′do-skop)—an instrument used to look directly into the bladder and urethra.
phlebolith (fleb′o-lith)—calcified or stony hard pieces within a vein.
presumptive diagnosis (pre-zump′tiv) (di-ag-no′sis)—a working diagnosis.
productive cough (pro-duk′tiv) (kawf)—a cough which produces phlegm, as opposed to a dry hacking cough.
prognosis (prog-no′sis)—outcome or future expectation of health.
prostatic (pros-tat′ik)—referring to the prostate.
pupil (pu′pil)—the opening in the center of the eye. (See Plate V, Appendix.)
pyelogram (pi′e-lo-gram)—a roentgenogram of the kidney and ureter.

R

resection (re-sek′shun)—excision or removal of tissue.
resectoscope (re-sek′to-skop)—an instrument used to resect tissue.

S

spinal anesthetic (spi′nal) (an-es-thet′ik)—anesthesia obtained by numbing the nerves issuing from the spinal cord.
splenomegaly (sple-no-meg′ah-le)—enlargement of the spleen.
sublingual (sub-ling′gual)—under the tongue.

T

testicular (tes-tik′u-lar)—referring to the testes or male gonads.
trabeculae (trah-bek′u-la)—thickened bands of muscle tissue.
transurethral (trans-u-re′thral)—traversing the urethra or via the urethra.
trigone (tri′gon)—the part of the urinary bladder nearest its outlet.
trilobar (tri-lo′bar)—having three lobes—here referring to the three lobes of the prostate.

U

ulcer (ul′ser)—an eroded or worn out area in tissue.
upper gastrointestinal series—a series of X-rays outlining the upper gastrointestinal tract.
ureterovesical junction (u-re-ter-o-ves′e-kal)—the point of joining of the ureter to the bladder.
urethral sounds (u-re′thral)—metal instruments graduated in size which are used to stretch or dilate the urethral passage.
urinary retention (u′ri-ner-e) (re-ten′shun)—inability to pass one's urine.

V

verumontanum (ve-ru-mon-ta′num)—a structure in the male urethra where the ejaculatory (seminal) ducts enter.
vesicle (ves′e-kal)—the urinary bladder. Also describes a blister (a fluid filled sac).
vesicle outlet obstruction—blockage to the outlet or passage from the urinary bladder.

Student: _____

Metropolitan Medical Center

HISTORY AND PHYSICAL EXAM

name hospital no.

address date of birth

  occupation

date race

physician room no.

Student: _____

Metropolitan Medical Center

X-RAY REPORT

name　　　　　　　　　　　　　　　　　　**hospital no.**

age　　　　　　　　　　　　　　　　　　　**x-ray no.**

sex　　　　　　　　　　　　　　　　　　　**room no.**

physician　　　　　　　　　　　　　　　　**date**

Student: _____

Metropolitan Medical Center
OPERATIVE RECORD

name

preoperative diagnosis

postoperative diagnosis

surgeon
second assistant

circulating nurse

operation title or
description

hospital no.

room no.

date

first assistant
instrument
nurse
sponge count

Student: _____

Metropolitan Medical Center

PATHOLOGY REPORT

name

tissue

date received

date reported

hospital no.

room no.

pathology
report no.

Student: _____

Metropolitan Medical Center

DISCHARGE SUMMARY

name hospital no.

admitted room no.

discharged age

diagnosis

surgery

complications

special procedures

consultations

135

WRITTEN QUIZ NO. 2

Name _____

Date _____

Score _____

SECTION I

Directions: In the Answers column write the appropriate word from the vocabulary list below that defines the statement.

axilla	colon	glycosuria	medulla
basilar	cystotomy	hypertrophy	stroma
cancer	dyspnea	isotope	subcutaneous
cervix	fibrosis	laparotomy	supine
cholesterol	gland	lumen	tympanotomy

	Answers	For Scoring
1. Underlying supportive tissue	_____	1. _____
2. Surgical exploration of the abdomen	_____	2. _____
3. Lying on one's back	_____	3. _____
4. Incision into the eardrum	_____	4. _____
5. The lowermost part of an organ	_____	5. _____
6. The armpit	_____	6. _____
7. Sugar in the urine	_____	7. _____
8. A general term for the large bowel	_____	8. _____
9. Scar tissue	_____	9. _____
10. A secreting organ	_____	10. _____
11. Under the skin	_____	11. _____
12. A fat-like substance of the blood	_____	12. _____
13. The interior space of a tube-like structure	_____	13. _____
14. A malignancy	_____	14. _____
15. Difficult breathing	_____	15. _____
16. Overgrowth of tissue	_____	16. _____
17. A radioactive tracer substance	_____	17. _____
18. A surgical opening into the urinary bladder	_____	18. _____
19. The neck of the womb	_____	19. _____
20. A soft marrow-like substance	_____	20. _____

SECTION II

Directions: In the Answers column write the numbers that correctly answer the question.

When blood pressure is dictated as "120 over 80," which is the systolic number and which is the diastolic number?

	Answers	For Scoring
1. Diastolic	_____	1. _____
2. Systolic	_____	2. _____

SECTION III

Directions: Name at least four organ systems included in the Review of Systems.

	For Scoring
1. _____	1. _____
2. _____	2. _____
3. _____	3. _____
4. _____	4. _____

CASE H

Student: _____

name Helen Hernandez

address 3460 Camellia Court
Chula Vista, CA 92011-3217

situation This very ill 30-year-old woman was admitted to the hospital with a history of abdominal complaints and jaundice. Ten days prior she had given birth to her fourth child. She underwent various X-ray studies as part of her evaluation to determine her illness. A consultant, a gastroenterologist, was asked to see the patient to help in diagnosis and management. Diagnosis was acute infectious hepatitis, an illness that is usually transmitted by oral ingestion of infected materials or by blood transfusion.

Plate II in the Appendix is related to this case.

sequence of reports

H-1
History and Physical Exam
Completed _____

H-2
X-ray Report
Completed _____

H-3
Consultant's Report
Completed _____

H-4
Discharge Summary
Completed _____

Note: Enter the date of completion for each report. When you have finished all the reports, tear this sheet out and give to your instructor along with the completed transcripts.

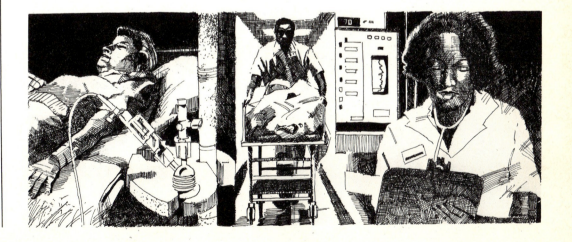

DEFINITIONS OF WORDS, PHRASES, AND ABBREVIATIONS

A

anemia (ah-ne'me-ah)—a condition characterized by a lack of or decrease in the red blood cells.
antiemetic (an-te-e-met'ik)—medication to combat nausea and vomiting.
antrum (an'trum)—an anatomical location in the stomach.
ascending colon—a specific part of the colon (large bowel) located in the right side of the abdomen.

B

barium (ba're-um)—a metallic element when mixed in solution is used to outline organs on X-ray.
bilirubin (bil-e-roo'bin)—a red bile pigment processed in the liver.
bruit (broot'); plural, **bruits** (broots')—an abnormal sound heard in an organ caused by impaired or abnormal blood flow.

C

capsule (kap'sul)—a small digestible case into which medication is placed.
carbohydrate (kar-bo-hi'drat)—a basic food substance, principally consisting of sugar and starches.
cesarean section (se-za're-an)—incision through the abdomen and uterus to deliver the fetus.
clavicle (klav'e-kl)—the collarbone. (See Plate III, Appendix.)
common bile duct (bil) (dukt)—the large duct transporting the bile from the liver to the intestine.
conception (kon-sep'shun)—successful fertilization of the egg.
consultation (kon-sul-ta'shun)—a deliberation among physicians regarding diagnosis and treatment.
contraceptives (kon-trah-sep'tivs)—measures designed to prevent pregnancy.
costal (kos'tal)—referring to the ribs.
costal margin (kos'tal) (mar'jin)—the lower margin of the rib cage.

D

debilitated (de-bil'li-ta-ted)—suffering from debility.
debility (de-bil'i-te)—a state of weakness and exhaustion.
delineate (de-lin'e-at); past tense, **delineated** (de-lin'e-a-ted)—to portray or diagram.
descending colon—a specific part of the colon (large bowel) located in the left side of the abdomen.
disoriented (dis-o're-en-ted)—confusion regarding one's surroundings, time, and place.
duodenal loop (du-o-de'nal) (loop)—the loop which the duodenum makes after it leaves the stomach.

E

elliptical (e-lip'ti-kal)—in the form or shape of an ellipse.
episiotomy (e-piz-e-ot'o-me)—an incision made in the birth canal to facilitate vaginal delivery of a baby.
exacerbation (eg-sas-er-ba'shun)—a worsening of one's condition or symptoms.
exophthalmos (ek-sof-thal'mus)—bulging eyeballs.

G

gallbladder (gawl'blad-der)—the organ which stores the bile produced by the liver. (See Plate II, Appendix.)
gastroenterology (gas-tro-en-ter-ol'-o-je)—devoted to the study of disease of the digestive tract.

H

hemolysis (he-mol'is-is)—the destruction or breaking up (lysis) of red blood cells.
hemolytic (he-mo-lit'ik)—pertaining to hemolysis.
hepatitis (hep-ah-ti'tis)—inflammation of the liver.

I

infectious (in-fek'shus)—contagious, capable of being transmitted from one subject to another by contact.

L

LDH—lactic dehydrogenase
leukopenia (lu-ko-pen'e-ah)—a decrease in the amount of white blood cells in the body.
lysis (li'sis)—dissolution, the gradual breakup of a disease process.

M

motility (mo-til'i-te)—movement or ability to move.

O

opacify (o-pas'i-fi); past tense, **opacified** (o-pas'i-fid)—here meaning to become a distinct shadow on X-ray film.

P

paravertebral (par-ah-ver'te-bral)—around or adjacent to the vertebrae.
parenteral (par-en'ter-al)—administered into the body by injection either into the muscle or into a vein.
phlebitis (fle-bi'tis)—inflammation of a vein or veins.
placenta (plah-sen'tah)—the organ within the womb from which the fetus receives nourishment from the mother.
placenta previa (plah-sen'tah) (pre'-ve-ah)—a condition in which the placenta is implanted in the lowermost part of the womb blocking the birth canal and normal exit of the baby.
postpartum (post-par'tum)—after delivery, following the birth of a child.

prescription (pre-skrip'shun)—a written direction for the dispensation of medication.
proctoscopy (prok-tos'ko-pe)—direct evaluation of the rectum with an examining instrument.
protein (pro'te-in)—a food substance found principally in meat and animal products.
pylorus (pi-lo'rus)—an anatomic area of the stomach at its junction with the small bowel.

R

reflux (re'fluks)—a backward flow.
regimen (rej'i-men)—a prescribed course of treatment.

S

sanguineous (sang-gwin'e-us)—relating to or containing blood.
scleral (skle'ral)—referring to the sclerae.
scout film—a preliminary X-ray taken of an organ to check for technique and background.
serosanguineous (se-ro-sang-gwin'-e-us)—composed of both serous and sanguineous components.
serous (se'rus)—relating to or containing serum.
SGOT—serum glutamic-oxalactic transaminase
SGPT—serum glutamic-pyruoic transaminase

sigmoidoscopy (sig-moid-os'ko-pe)—direct evaluation of the sigmoid colon with a sigmoidoscope.
subcostal (sub-kos'tal)—below the ribs.
supraclavicular (su-prah-klah-vik'u-lar)—above the clavicle (collarbone).

T

tachypnea (tak-ip'-ne-ah)—rapid respirations or breathing.
transfusions (trans-fu'zhunz)—administration of blood to the patient intravenously.
transverse colon—a specific part of the colon (large bowel) located in the right side of the abdomen.

Student: _____

Metropolitan Medical Center

HISTORY AND PHYSICAL EXAM

name   hospital no.

address   date of birth

                                                occupation

date   race

physician   room no.

Student: _____

Metropolitan Medical Center

X-RAY REPORT

name												hospital no.

age												x-ray no.

sex												room no.

physician												date

Student: _____

Metropolitan Medical Center

CONSULTANT'S REPORT

to						hospital no.

from						room no.

re						date

reason for consultation

Student: _____

Metropolitan Medical Center

DISCHARGE SUMMARY

name   hospital no.

admitted   room no.

discharged   age

diagnosis

surgery

complications

special procedures

consultations

CASE I

Student: _____

name Izumi, Ishida

address 5917 University Avenue
San Diego, Ca 92115-0976

situation This 56-year-old woman with a lengthy history of prior medical problems was admitted quite ill with symptoms of fever, weakness, headache, and cough. Her evaluation in addition to X-ray studies included an examination of her lower bowel during which an abnormal growth, a polyp of the colon, was removed surgically. The pathology report indicated this growth to be benign. Her major illness was diagnosed as an acute infection involving the heart valves, bacterial endocarditis, and appropriate treatment was undertaken. Her hospital course and therapy are outlined in the discharge summary.

The specialty that deals with the study of the heart and its functions is cardiology, another branch of internal medicine. You will recall that diseases of the digestive system are treated by a gastroenterologist, also a branch of internal medicine.

The following Plates are related to this case: Plates II and VIII.

sequence of reports

I-1
History and Physical Exam
Completed _____

I-2
X-ray Report
Completed _____

I-3
Operative Record
Completed _____

I-4
Pathology Report
Completed _____

I-5
Discharge Summary
Completed _____

Note: Enter the date of completion for each report. When you have finished all the reports, tear this sheet out and give to your instructor along with the completed transcripts.

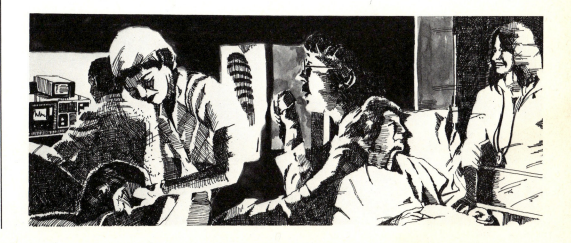

151

Complete the written quiz on page 167 before submitting your work for this case. Follow the directions of your instructor for checking your answers.

DEFINITIONS OF WORDS, PHRASES, AND ABBREVIATIONS

A

acholic (a-kol'ik)—without bile.
alopecia (al-o-pe'she-ah)—loss of hair.
aneurysm (an'u-rizm)—a sac-like blowout area in an artery.
antecubital (an-te-ku'be-tal)—the area in front of the elbow.
anterolaterally (an-te-ro-lat'er-a-le)—extending from an area in front of the body to one side or the other.
antihypertensive drugs (an-te-hi-per-ten'siv)—drugs used in the treatment of hypertension or high blood pressure.
aorta (a-or'tah)—the main artery in the body leading from the heart to various organs. (See Plate VIII, Appendix.)
aortic (a-or'tik)—referring to the aorta.
aortic insufficiency—insufficiency or malfunction of the aortic heart valve.
arthrotomy (ar-throt'o-me)—an operation in which a joint space is surgically entered and explored.
ascites (ah-si'tez)—accumulation of fluid in the abdominal cavity.
asymptomatic (a-simp-to-mat'ik)—without symptoms.
ataxia (a-tak'se-ah)—staggering, loss of balance.
atheroma (ath-er-o'mah)—fat deposit(s) within the lumen of an artery.
atheromatous (ath-er-o'mah-tus)—having many and significant atheroma causing disease.
atrium (a'tre-um)—a small heart chamber. (See Plate VIII, Appendix.)
atypical (a-tip'e-kal)—abnormal, not true to the usual form.

B

bacterial (bak-te're-al)—referring to or caused by bacteria.
basement membrane (bas'ment) (mem'bran)—a thin layer of cells interposed between epithelium and connective tissue.
bibasilar (bi-bas'i-lar)—in both basal areas.
biopsy (bi'op-se)—the removal of a piece of tissue or piece of an organ for microscopic examination to determine the nature and extent of disease in that organ.
bitemporal (bi-tem'po-ral)—in both temporal areas.
bowel (bow'el)—a general term for the intestine.
buccal (buk'al)—pertaining to the cheek.
buccal membrane (buk'al) (mem'bran)—the inner lining of the cheek.

C

carcinoma (kar-si-no'mah)—cancer or a malignant condition.
cardiotonic (kar-de-o-ton'ik)—drugs, treatment, and the like which have a stimulating, supportive, or tonic effect on the heart.
cartilage (kar'ti-lij)—the firm, tough, connective tissue between bone surfaces, gristle.
cataract (kat'ah-rakt)—a cloudiness of the lens of the eye leading to loss of vision.
cauda equina (kaw'dah) (e-kwin'ah)—long nerve roots issuing from the very end of the spinal cord having the appearance of a horse's tail.
cephalalgia (sef-ah-lal'je-ah)—headache.
chemotherapy (ke-mo-ther'ah-pe)—treatment with specific drugs, anticancer drugs.
clonus (klo'nus)—a rapid series of alternating contraction and relaxation of a muscle or group of muscles about an extremity.
coarctation (ko-ark-ta'shun)—an abnormal narrowing of an artery causing obstruction to the flow of blood past this narrowing.
columnar (ko-lum'nar)—describes cells which are tall and column-like.
compression (kom-presh'un)—the act or state of being squeezed together.
compression fracture (kom-presh'un) (frak'tur)—a break in a bone characteristically showing the two broken parts being squeezed into or onto one another.
congestive heart failure (kon-jes'tiv)—failure of the heart to effectively pump blood, thus causing a congestion or back up of fluid in various organs.
cornea (kor'ne-ah)—the transparent outer covering of the pupil of the eye. (See Plate V, Appendix.)
cuboidal (ku-boid'al)—describes cells which are small and cube-like.
cyst (sist)—a soft fluid-filled sac of tissue.
cystic (sis'tik)—being cyst-like or soft and fluid-filled.
cystourethrocele (sis-to-u-re'thro-sel)—a condition caused by a lack of support to the urinary bladder and urethra in the female.

D

diaphoresis (di-ah-fo-re'sis)—profuse sweating.
diaphoretic (di-ah-fo-ret'ik)—being in a state of diaphoresis.
Dilantin (di-lan'ten)—a brand name drug used in the treatment of epilepsy.
diplopia (dip-lo'pe-ah)—double vision.
diuretic (di-u-ret'ik)—drugs which increase the amount of urine excreted from the body.
dura (du'rah)—the strong fibrous tissue sheath covering the spinal cord.
dysarthria (dis-ar'thre-ah)—difficulty speaking, especially in articulation or forming words.

E

endocarditis (en-do-kar-di'tis)—an inflammation of the inner lining of the heart muscle or heart valves.
enteritis (en-ter-i'tis)—nonspecific inflammation of the gastrointestinal tract.
epiglottis (ep-e-glot'is)—a saddle shaped piece of tissue situated deep in the throat, which folds down over the windpipe in the act of swallowing so that food or liquid cannot enter the lungs. (See Plates I, VI, Appendix.)

epilepsy (ep'e-lep-se)—a condition characterized by the occurrence of seizures or fits.
epistaxis (ep-e-stak'sis)—bleeding from the nose, a bloody nose.
erosion (e-ro'zhun)—a wearing away of tissue, an ulceration.
etiology (e-te-ol'o-je)—the cause or causative factor.
excisional (ek-sizh'un-al)—referring to excision.
excoriation (eks-ko-re-a'shun)—a scratch mark or marks.
exogenous (eks-oj'e-nus)—originating from or produced outside the body.
exostosis (ek-sos-to'sis)—a bony prominence or knob.
extradural (eks-trah-du'ral)—outside (extra) the dura.

F

fibrocystic disease (fi-bro-sis'tik)—a disease process of the breasts or other organs composed of numerous small cysts and scar tissue.
fifth lumbar vertebra (lum'bar) (ver'te-brah)—the fifth or last vertebra in the lumbar area low in the back.
flatplate—an X-ray of the abdomen taken with the patient supine.
fleshy—soft and flesh-like as opposed to hard and gristle-like.
flexion (flek'shun)—bending of a joint to bring the two bones it connects together.
fluoroscope (floo-o'ro-skop)—an X-ray machine which can produce instant images of the interior of the body.
fluoroscopy (floo-or-os'ko-pe)—the act of using the fluoroscope to examine the patient.
fulgurate (ful'gu-rat)—to cauterize or destroy tissue by burning.

G

genitalia (jen-e-ta'le-ah)—the male or female external genital organs.
gluteal region (gloo'te-al)—the buttocks.

H

hepatorenal (hep-ah-to-re'nal)—refers to both the liver and the kidney.
hyperchromatism (hi-per-kro'mah-tizm)—excessive pigmentation.
hypotonia (hi-po-to'ne-ah)—decrease of, or diminution in, strength or power.

I

indirect laryngoscopy (lar-ing-gos'-ko-pe)—examination of the larynx done with mirrors.
interspace (in'ter-spas)—the space between any two vertebrae, joints, or other organs.
intracranial (in-trah-kra'ne-al)—within (intra) the cranium or skull.
intramuscularly (in-trah-mus'ku-lar-le)—within (intra) or into the muscle.
invasion (in-va'zhun)—extension into surrounding areas.

J

JVP (jugular venous pulse)—pulsation seen or felt over the juglar vein.

L

L3, L4, L5—third, fourth, and fifth lumbar vertebrae.
labium majora (la'be-um) (mah-jo'rah)—the external or large lip of the female genitalia.
laryngoscopy (lar-ing-gos'ko-pe)—examination of the larynx.
larynx (lar'inks)—the voice box. (See Plates I, VI, Appendix.)
leukoplakia (lu-ko-pla'ke-ah)—an abnormal thickening (whitish in color) of lining tissue.
lordosis (lor-do'sis)—abnormal or accentuated curvature of the spine, saddle back.

M

maculopapular (mak-u-lo-pap'u-lar)—a skin rash which is both red and angry looking and composed of raised bumps on the skin.
mammography (mam-og'rah-fe)—special X-ray examination of the breasts.
metastasis (me-tas'tah-sis); plural, **metastases** (me-tas'tah-ses)—the spread of a malignant disease.
metastatic (met-ah-stat'ik)—a cancer that spreads outside of the organ in which it develops.
migraine (mi'gran)—a severe type of headache.
mucin (mu'sin)—a thick liquid substance produced by certain cells.
myelogram (mi'el-o-gram)—a specialized X-ray study wherein contrast material (dye) is injected into the spinal canal to study its shape, contour, and patency.
myxedema (mik-se-de'mah)—a disease state caused by under activity of the thyroid gland.

N

necrosis (ne-kro'sis)—death of tissue.
nephritis (ne-fri'tis)—a general term for inflammation of the kidneys.
nephropathy (nef-rop'ah-the)—any disease of the kidneys.
nephrotoxic (nef-ro-tok'sik)—harmful or toxic to the kidneys.
neurological (nu-ro-loj'e-kal)—pertaining to the nervous system.
nevus (ne'vus)—a skin mole.
nucleus (nu'kle-us); plural, **nuclei** (nu'kle-i)—the central portion of a cell containing dark staining material called chromatin.

O

obese (o-bes')—overweight, fat.
obesity (o-bes'i-te)—the state of being fat.
obstipation (ob-sti-pa'shun)—severe constipation, blockage of the passage of digested material through the intestinal tract.

P

pancreas (pan'kre-as)—the organ which produces insulin and other substances which aid digestion. (See Plate II, Appendix.)

papillary (pap′i-ler-e)—referring to a small nipple-like projection of an organ.
papilledema (pap-i-le-de′mah)—swelling of the optic disk (that part of the eye where the veins and blood vessels enter).
paralysis (pah-ral′is-is)—loss of movement or power in a muscle or limb.
parametrial (par-ah-me′tre-al)—referring to the parametrium.
parametrium (par-ah-me′tre-um)—the connective tissue within the female pelvis extending from the womb to the side walls of the pelvis.
paresis (pah-re′sis) or (par′e-sis)—partial or incomplete paralysis.
pedunculated (pe-dung′ku-lat-ed)—a structure having a stalk or sitting on the end of a stalk.
pericardial (per-e-kar′de-al)—the area immediately around the heart.
phenobarbital (fe-no-bar′bi-tal)—a sedative drug used also in epilepsy.
pigmented (pig′ment-ed)—containing pigment or dark coloring material.
pneumonia (nu-mo′ne-ah)—an inflammation of the lungs.
projections (pro-jek′shuns)—the projected image of the X-ray onto film.
pruritus (proo-ri′tis)—itching.
ptosis (to′sis)—drooping or sagging.
pyelonephritis (pi-el-o-ne-fri′tis)—a bacterial infection of the kidney.

R

radiation therapy (ra-de-a′shun) (ther′ah-pe)—treatment with X-rays to help stop the spread of cancer.
recrudescence (re-kroo-des′ens)—the recurrence of a symptom or disease after a temporary relief, a relapse.
regurgitation (re-gur-ji-ta′shun)—a backward flow.
retina (ret′i-nah)—a specialized part of the eye in the inner aspect, which is responsible for the perception of light and color. (See Plate V, Appendix.)

S

scapula (skap′u-lah)—the shoulder blade.
sedation (se-da′shun)—the act of making calm or administering a calming drug.
snare loop—a special cutting wire in the shape of a loop which can snare tissue and cut if off.
stalk (stawk)—a narrow connection from one structure to another.
sternum (ster′num)—the breast bone. (See Plate III, Appendix.)
stool (stool)—passed fecal material.
strabismus (strah-biz′mus)—an abnormal deviation of the eyeball.
subacute (sub-ah-kut′)—less than acute, used to characterize a disease which is not fully evident or easily detected.
substernal (sub-ster′nal)—beneath or under the sternum.
sulfa drugs (sul′fah)—medication made from sulfa, frequently used in urinary tract infections.
sympathectomy (sim-pah-thek′to-me)—an operation done in the treatment of hypertension, where various sympathetic nerves are cut.
sympathetic nerves (sim-pah-thet′ik) (nervz)—the nerves that regulate the automatic processes of body function over which we exercise no conscious control, such as heart action, release of digestive juices, and control of blood pressure.
syndrome (sin′drom)—the composite of various specific signs and symptoms constituting together the picture of a disease.

T

T11—thoracic vertebra, 11th.
temporal (tem′po-ral)—the temporal bone area of the skull, the area to the sides and just above the ear. (See Plate VII, Appendix.)
tinnitus (tin-i′tus)—ringing in the ears.
transient (tran′shent)—fleeting or temporary, coming and going.
turgor (tur′gor)—fullness or resiliency.

V

vertebra (ver′te-brah); plural, **vertebrae** (ver′te-bra)—the back bones of the spine extending from the head to the tail bone. They are divided and numbered according to anatomical areas. (See Plate III, Appendix.)
vulva (vul′vah)—the external aspect of the female genitalia.

W

wheeze (hwez)—the noise made by air passing through a narrowed respiratory passage where breathing is difficult.

Student: _____

Metropolitan Medical Center

HISTORY AND PHYSICAL EXAM

name							hospital no.

address							date of birth

							occupation

date							race

physician							room no.

Student: _____

Metropolitan Medical Center

X-RAY REPORT

name   hospital no.

age   x-ray no.

sex   room no.

physician   date

Student: _____

Metropolitan Medical Center

OPERATIVE RECORD

name   **hospital no.**

preoperative diagnosis   **room no.**

                                                                         date

postoperative diagnosis

                                                                         first assistant
                                                                         instrument
                        surgeon   **nurse**
                        second assistant   **sponge count**

                        circulating nurse

                        operation title or
                        description

161

Student: _____

Metropolitan Medical Center

PATHOLOGY REPORT

name

tissue

date received

date reported

hospital no.

room no.

pathology
report no.

Student: _____

Metropolitan Medical Center

DISCHARGE SUMMARY

name hospital no.

admitted room no.

discharged age

diagnosis

surgery

complications

special procedures

consultations

WRITTEN QUIZ NO. 3

Name _____

Date _____

Score _____

SECTION I

Directions: In the Answers column write the appropriate word from the vocabulary list below that defines the statement.

alopecia	bilirubin	costal	hepatitis
anulus	biopsy	diaphoresis	ileum
aorta	bronchus	enuresis	paresis
asthma	buccal	epistaxis	pruritus
atypical	chemotherapy	friable	ptosis
aural	clavicle	fulgurate	recrudescence
			tachypnea

                                                                             Answers   **For Scoring**

1. Inflammation of the liver .... _____ 1. _____
2. The collarbone .... _____ 2. _____
3. Rapid respiration .... _____ 3. _____
4. Loss of hair .... _____ 4. _____
5. Bed wetting .... _____ 5. _____
6. Referring to the ribs .... _____ 6. _____
7. An air tube in the lung .... _____ 7. _____
8. Itching .... _____ 8. _____
9. Profuse sweating .... _____ 9. _____
10. A condition characterized by wheezing and gasping .... _____ 10. _____
11. To cauterize .... _____ 11. _____
12. A drug treatment .... _____ 12. _____
13. A part of the small bowel .... _____ 13. _____
14. Removal of tissues for examination .... _____ 14. _____
15. Bleeding from the nose .... _____ 15. _____
16. Abnormal .... _____ 16. _____
17. A red bile pigment processed in the liver .... _____ 17. _____
18. Drooping or sagging .... _____ 18. _____
19. Relating to the ear .... _____ 19. _____

20. The main artery in the body .... _____ 20. _____
21. A relapse .... _____ 21. _____
22. Bleeding easily .... _____ 22. _____
23. Referring to the cheek .... _____ 23. _____
24. Partial paralysis .... _____ 24. _____
25. A ring or ring-shaped structure .... _____ 25. _____

SECTION II

Directions: In the Answers column write the word or words that correctly complete the statement.

The X-ray Department of a hospital performs routine X-rays such as bone X-rays, abdominal X-rays, and chest X-rays. Special tests of internal organs by introducing contrast material into the body are also performed. Name three such tests that you have encountered in the cases you have studied.

For Scoring

1. _____ 1. _____
2. _____ 2. _____
3. _____ 3. _____

SECTION III

Directions: In the Answers column write the word or words that correctly answer the question.

What organ, organs, or cavities are examined with the following:

	Answers	For Scoring
1. Ophthalmoscope	_____	1. _____
2. Cystoscope	_____	2. _____
3. Sigmoidoscope	_____	3. _____
4. Laparoscope	_____	4. _____

CASE J

Student: _____

name John K. Jenkins

address 1682 Sloane Street
National City, CA 92050-4007

situation This 64-year-old male was admitted to the hospital for treatment of liver disease secondary to chronic alcoholism. His admission history and physical exam indicated severe liver dysfunction in a severely ill patient. X-ray studies confirmed the diagnosis, cirrhosis, and degree of involvement. Cirrhosis is marked by degeneration of the liver cells. The patient's condition worsened and, in spite of therapy, he died of his disease while in the hospital. An autopsy was performed.

An autopsy is performed by a pathologist to determine the actual cause of death. Unless it is demanded by a public authority, an autopsy cannot be performed without permission of the next of kin.

Plate II relates to this case.

sequence of reports

J-1
History and Physical Exam
Completed _____

J-2
X-ray Report
Completed _____

J-3
Autopsy Report
Completed _____

Note: Enter the date of completion for each report. When you have finished all the reports, tear this sheet out and give to your instructor along with the completed transcripts.

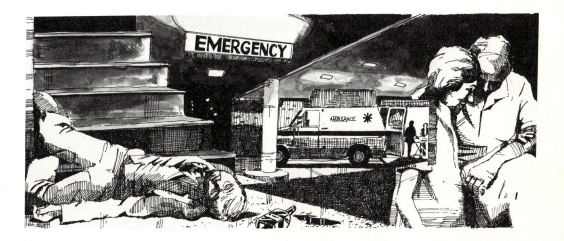

Transcribe Cassette Quiz No. 3 on the form on page 179 after completing work on Case J.

DEFINITIONS OF WORDS, PHRASES, AND ABBREVIATIONS

A

adenocarcinoma (ad-e-no-kar-si-no'mah)—a common type of cancer.
adrenal (ad-re'nal)—a gland of internal secretion situated above the kidney, one on each side.
alcoholism (al'ko-hol-izm)—a disease characterized by excessive drinking of alcoholic beverages.
alkaline phosphatase (al'kah-lin) (fos'fah-tas)—a specific enzyme present in liver and bony tissue.
alveolus (al-ve'o-lus); plural, **alveoli** (al-ve'o-li)—a small air sac in the lung.
ambulatory (am'bu-la-to-re)—upright and walking.
ammonia (ah-mo'ne-ah)—a blood constituent present normally in trace amounts, but increased in severe liver disease.
autopsy (aw'top-se)—an examination of the body, external and internal, made after death (postmortem).

B

bile ducts (bil) (dukts)—these are small channels or ducts within the liver that transport bile to the gallbladder.
bloating (blot'ing)—a feeling of fullness.

C

cholestasis (ko-le-sta'sis)—a stoppage in the flow of bile.
cirrhosis (sir-o'sis)—a disease characterized by replacement of normal tissue with scar tissue.
coronary (kor'o-na-re)—referring to the heart.
cortex (kor'teks)—the outermost fleshy part of the kidney or any internal organ.
croup (kroop)—characterized by resonant barking cough, hoarseness, and persistent high-pitched respiratory sound.
croupy (kroop'e)—referring to the croup.

D

decompensated (de-kom'pen-sa-ted)—suffering from decompensation.
decongestant (de-kon-jes'tant)—a medication designed to relieve the congestion or stuffiness of a head cold and/or cough.
demise (de-miz')—death, expiration.
dermatologist (der-mah-tol'o-jist)—a physician who specializes in dermatology.
dermatology (der-mah-tol'o-je)—science dealing with the diagnosis and treatment of skin disease.
despondency (de-spon'den-se)—a feeling of severe mental depression.
differentiated (dif-er-en'-she-a-ted)—recognizable as containing specific and separate cells of a particular type.
digit (dij'it)—a finger or toe.
diphtheria (dif-the're-ah)—infectious disease of the throat causing difficult breathing.
dysfunction (dis-funk'shun)—abnormal function or operation of an organ.

E

ecchymosis (ek-e-mo'sis); plural, **ecchymoses** (ek-e-mo'ses)—a bruise, a black and blue mark.
ecchymotic (ek-e-mot'ik)—referring to an ecchymosis, or having ecchymoses.
eczema (ek'ze-mah)—a skin disease characterized by scaling and crusting of the skin.
emaciated (e-ma'-se-a-ted)—wasted away, having the appearance of loss of flesh and substance.
engorged (en-gorjd')—filled with blood.
enterocolitis (en-ter-o-ko-li'tis)—a nonspecific inflammation of the intestines.
enzyme (en'zim)—a substance secreted by cells that acts to enhance, produce, or speed up a specific chemical reaction in the body.
esophageal (e-sof-ah-je'al)—referring to the esophagus.
esophagus (e-sof'ah-gus)—the tube that carries food or liquid from the throat to the stomach. (See Plate VI, Appendix.)

F

fibrotic (fi-brot'ik)—having fibrosis or scarring.
fingerbreadths (fing'ger) (bredths')—the span of the examiner's fingers is often used to describe length of measurement of an organ or its enlargement.
follicles (fol'e-klz)—small skin pockets or glands.
frontal lobe (fron'tal) (lob)—a prominent part or lobe of brain tissue located in the front portion of the head (in the forehead). (See Plate VII, Appendix.)

G

glomerulus (glo-mer'u-lus); plural, **glomeruli** (glo-mer'u-li)—filtering component of the kidney.
granular (gran'u-lar)—grainy in consistency.
greater trochanter (tro-kan'ter)—the larger bony process or knob situated on the upper outside aspect of the femur.
gynecomastia (jin-e-ko-mas'te-ah)—abnormal enlargement of the breast in a male.

H

hepatic (he-pat'ik)—referring to the liver.
hiatal (hi-a'tal)—referring to a hiatus.
hiatal hernia (hi-a'tal) (her'ne-ah)—a protrusion of the stomach up into the chest cavity through an abnormal enlargement of the diaphragm, which separates both body cavities.
hiatus (hi-a'tus)—any gap or opening.
hyperemesis (hi-per-em'e-sis)—excessive vomiting.

hyperreflexia (hi-per-re-flek′se-ah) —exaggeration of reflexes.

I

icteric (ik-ter′ik)—jaundiced, colored yellow.
iris (i′ris); plural, **irides** (i′rid-ez)— that part of the pupil of the eye which is colored. (See Plate V, Appendix.)

J

jaundiced (jawn′dist)—having jaundice.

L

labile (la′bil)—unstable.
livor mortis (li′vor) (mor′tis)—the discoloration of the skin seen in dependent parts of the body after death.
lucent (lu′sent)—translucent, transmitting light.

M

meatal (me-a′tal)—referring to the meatus.
medial (me′de-al)—extending toward the middle or midline of the body or of an organ.
mediastinum (me-de-as-ti′num)—the middle part of the chest cavity dividing the right and left sides.
microgram (mi′kro-gram)—one millionth part of a gram.
microscopic (mi-kro-skop′ik)—referring to an extremely small size scale, visible only under the microscope.
mitosis (mi-to′sis)—the activity by which a cell divides and duplicates itself.

N

neuritis (nu-ri′tis)—an inflammation of a nerve or group of nerves.
nodular (nod′u-lar)—having many small bumps or nodules.
nodule (nod′ul)—a small prominence or bump which is solid and may be detected by touch.

O

occiput (ok′si-put)—the back of the head.

ostium (os′te-um); plural, **ostia** (os′te-ah)—an opening into a blood vessel or organ.

P

paroxysmal (par-ok-siz′mal)—occurring unpredictably and abruptly (without warning).
patent (pa′tent)—open, not blocked.
per high-powered field—the examination of tissue or fluid under a microscope; descriptions or numbers of cells seen in the average high-powered field.
periosteal (per-e-os′te-al)—referring to the periosteum.
periosteum (per-e-os′te-um)—the thin connective tissue covering a bone.
peripheral neuritis (peh-rif′er-al) (nu-ri′tis)—an inflammation of the nerves of the limbs.
pertussis (per-tus′is)—whooping cough.
pitting edema (e-de′mah)—edema which pits or indents when pushed or compressed by the examiner's finger.
pleomorphism (ple-o-mor′fism)— having varied and irregular shape.
proprioception (pro-pre-o-sep′shun) —the specific sensory awareness that makes us cognizant of attitude, movement, or shifting in position.
prosthesis (pros′the-sis)—a manufactured substitute for a body part, such as a limb or eye.
prosthetic (pros-thet′ik)—referring to being a prosthesis or a manufactured substitute.
protuberant (pro-tu′ber-ant)—projecting out.
psychiatrist (si-ki′ah-trist)—a physician who deals with the diagnosis and treatment of mental disorders.

R

RBC—red blood cells
resuscitate (re-sus′i-tat)—to revive or bring back to life.
resuscitative (re-sus-i-ta-tiv)—referring to the verb resuscitate.
Romberg test (rom′berg)—a test of balance.

rigor mortis (ri′gor) (mor′tis)— stiffening of the body occurring 1 to 7 hours after death.
Rinne test (ren′e)—an ear test to determine its function.
roentgen (rent′gen)—the international unit of x radiation, an X-ray.

S

seborrhea (seb-o-re′ah)—dandruff.
sediment (sed′i-ment)—material that sinks to the bottom of a liquid.
seizure (se′zhur)—a fit or convulsion.
sensorium (sen-so′re-um)—the patient's awareness, degree of orientation, and comprehension.
shifting dullness—a specific diagnostic sign of dullness perceived on percussion of the abdomen.
stenosis (ste-no′sis)—an abnormal constriction or narrowing.
syncope (sin′ko-pe)—fainting or a fainting spell.

T

trapezius muscles (trah-pe′ze-us)—the muscles of the back of the neck and shoulder.
tricuspid (tri-kus′pid)—having three points.
trochanter (tro-kan′ter)—a bony process or knob on the femur or thigh bone.
tubules (tu′bulz)—small tubes.
tumor (tu′mor)—an abnormal growth of tissue.
turbinate (tur′bi-nat)—inner cylindrical structure of the nose, a part of the breathing passage.

V

varices (var′i-sez)—another term for varicose veins.
visceromegaly (vis-er-o-meg′a-le) —enlargement of any viscus (any soft organ of the body as opposed to bone or muscle).

W

white matter—an anatomic subdivision of brain tissue.

Student: _____

Metropolitan Medical Center

HISTORY AND PHYSICAL EXAM

name	hospital no.
address	date of birth
	occupation
date	race
physician	room no.

Student: _____

Metropolitan Medical Center

X-RAY REPORT

name   hospital no.

age   x-ray no.

sex   room no.

physician   date

Student: _____

Metropolitan Medical Center

AUTOPSY REPORT

name

physician

hospital no.

room no.

pathology
report no.

Cassette Quiz No. 3   Student: _____

Metropolitan Medical Center

HISTORY AND PHYSICAL EXAM

name　　　　　　　　　　　　　　　　　　　　　　　　　**hospital no.**

address　　　　　　　　　　　　　　　　　　　　　　　　**date of birth**

　　　　　　　　　　　　　　　　　　　　　　　　　　　　　occupation

date　　　　　　　　　　　　　　　　　　　　　　　　　　**race**

physician　　　　　　　　　　　　　　　　　　　　　　　**room no.**

PLATE I
THE LUNGS AND AIR PASSAGES

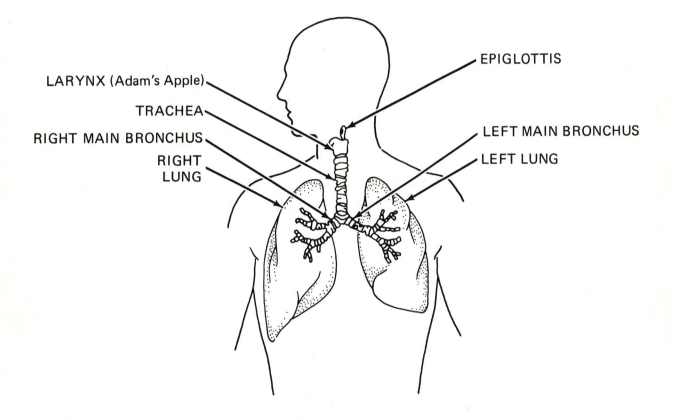

PLATE II
THORAX AND ABDOMEN

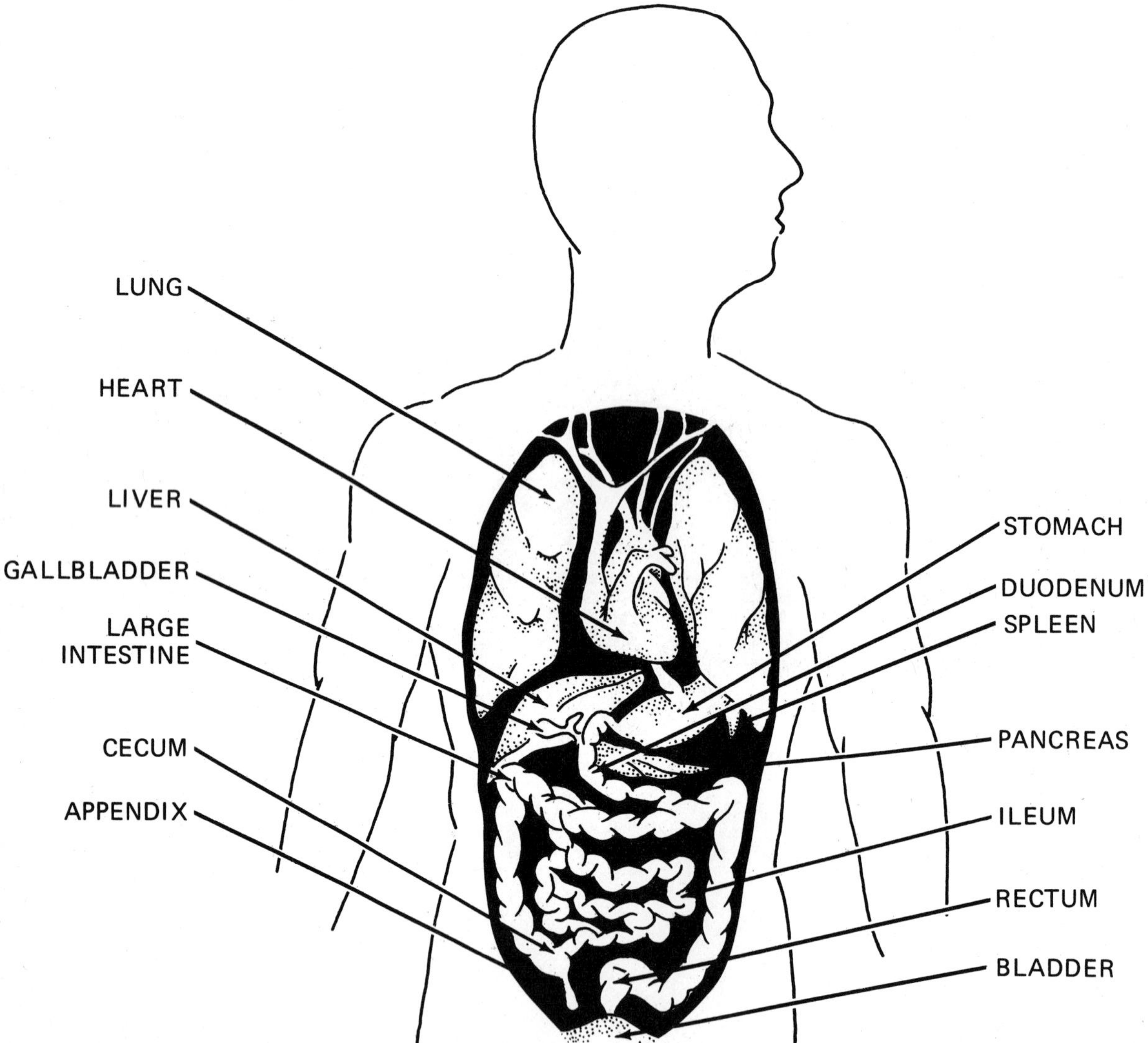

- LUNG
- HEART
- LIVER
- GALLBLADDER
- LARGE INTESTINE
- CECUM
- APPENDIX
- STOMACH
- DUODENUM
- SPLEEN
- PANCREAS
- ILEUM
- RECTUM
- BLADDER

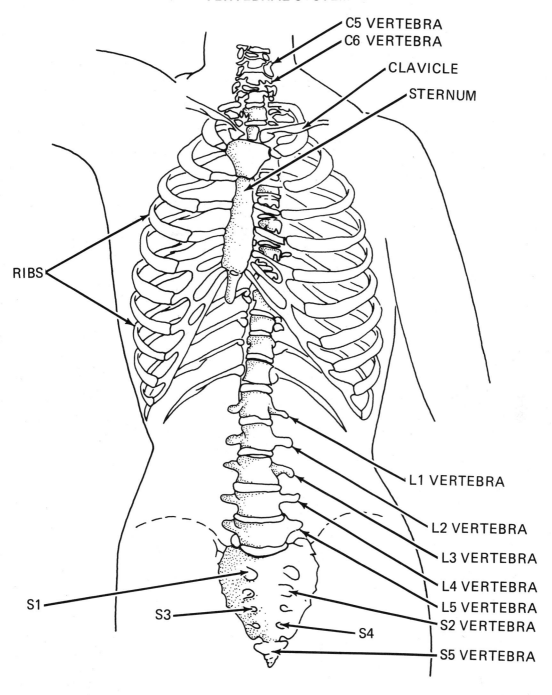

PLATE IV
EXTREMETIES

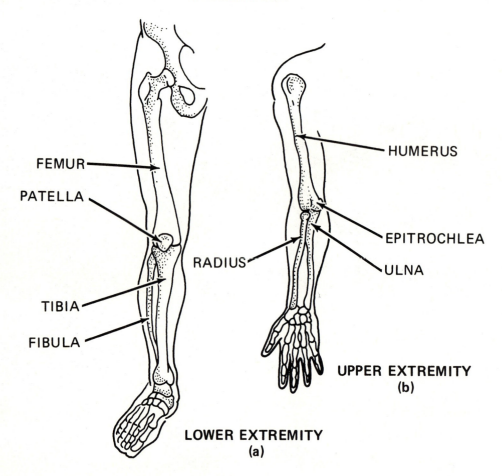

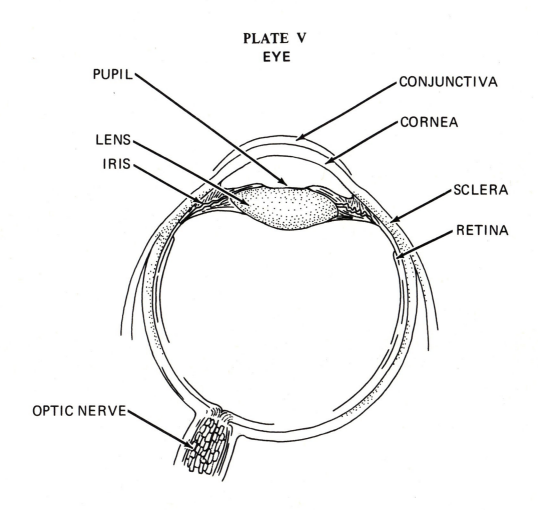

PLATE VI
UPPER RESPIRATORY TRACT AND ESOPHAGUS

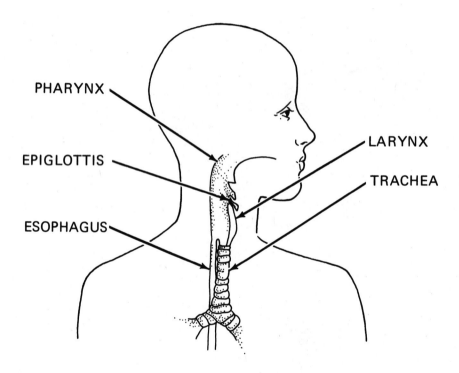

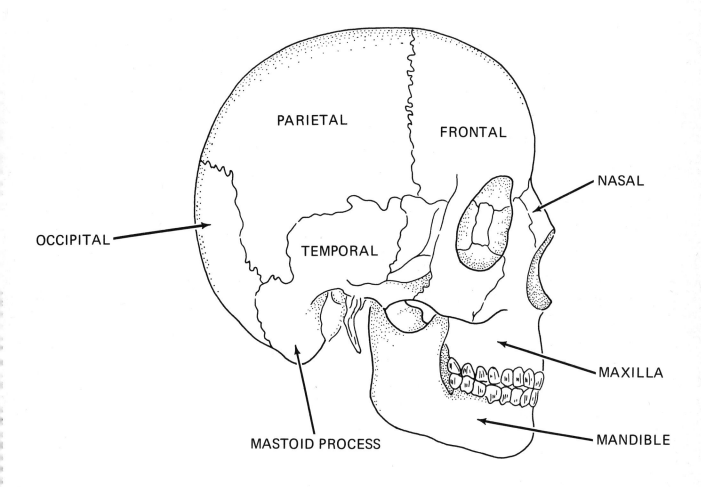

PLATE VIII
HEART AND ITS CHAMBERS

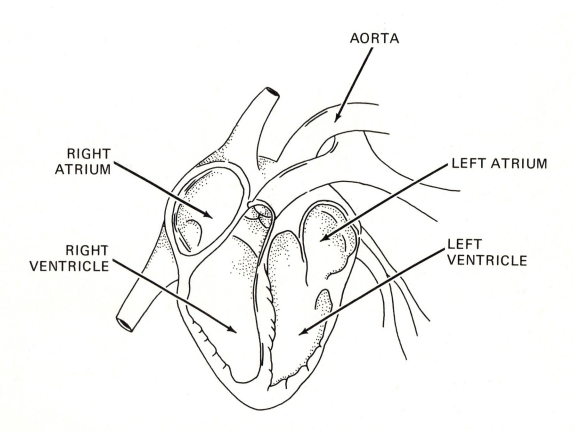

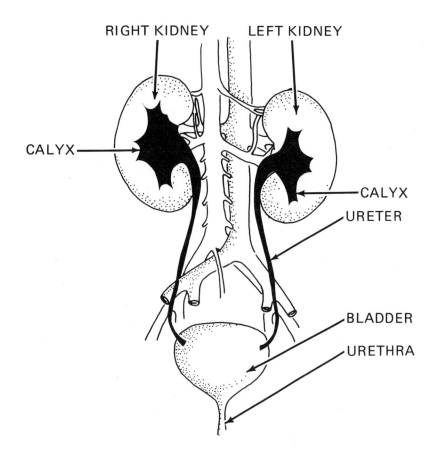

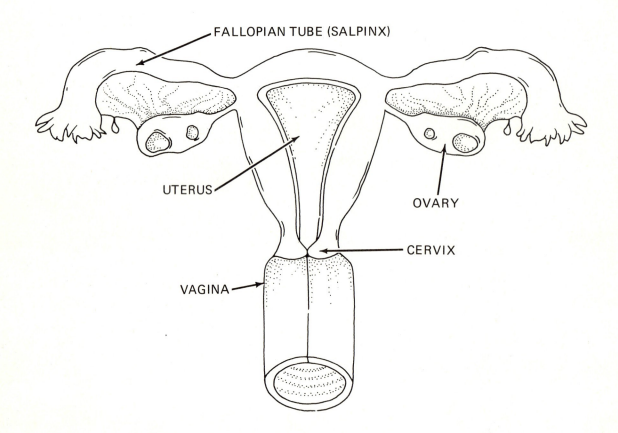

PLATE X
INTERNAL GENITAL ORGANS OF FEMALE

PLATE XI
STRUCTURE OF THE EAR

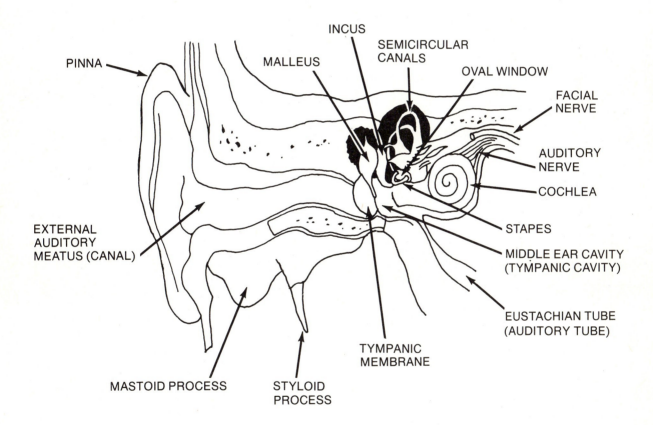

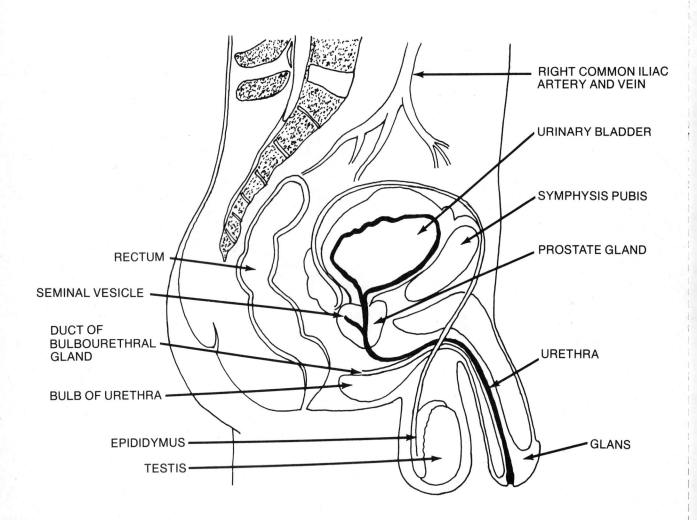

INDEX OF WORDS, PHRASES, AND ABBREVIATIONS

A

abortio (a-bor'shi-o) Case A
abscess (ab'ses) Case A
accommodation (ah-kom-o-da'shun) Case A
acetone (as'e-ton) Case B
acholic (a-kol'ik) Case I
adenitis (ad-eh-ni'tis) Case A
adenocarcinoma (ad-e-no-kar-si-no'mah) Case J
adenoidal (ad-e-noid'al) Case F
adenoids (ad'e-noidz) Case F
adenoma (ad-e-no'mah) Case G
adenopathy (ad-e-nop'ah-the) Case A
adhesions (ad-he'zhunz) Case F
adnexa (ad-nek'sa) Case A
adrenal (ad-re'nal) Case J
adrenalin (ad-ren'al-in) Case F
afebrile (a-feb'ril) Case B
air-fluid levels Case D
alcoholism (al'ko-hol-izm) Case J
alkaline phosphatase (al'kah-lin) (fos'fah-tas) Case J
alopecia (al-o-pe'she-ah) Case I
alveolus (al-ve'o-lus); plural, **alveoli** (al-ve'o-li) Case J
ambulate (am'bu-lat) Case D
ambulatory (am'bu-la-to-re) Case J
ammonia (ah-mo'ne-ah) Case J
Ampicillin (am-pi-si'lin) Case B
ampulla (am-pul'ah) Case G
anal (a'nal) Case B
analgesic (an-al-je'zik) Case C
anemia (ah-ne'me-ah) Case H
anesthesia (an-es-the'ze-ah) Case A
aneurysm (an'u-rizm) Case I
angina (an'jin-ah) Case C
angulated (ang'gu-lat-ed) Case E
anorexia (an-o-rek'se-ah) Case A
anorexic (an-o-rek'sik) Case D
antecubital (an-te-ku'be-tal) Case I
anterior (an-te're-or) Case C
anteriorly (an-te're-or-le) Case F
anterolaterally (an-te-ro-lat'er-a-le) Case I
anteroposterior (an'ter-o-pos-ter'e-or) Case C
anteverted (an-te-vert'ed) Case D
antibiotic (an-te-bi-ot'ik) Case B
anticholinergics (an-te-ko-lin-er'jikz) Case G
anticoagulant (an-te-ko-ag'u-lant) Case C
antiemetic (an-te-e-met'ik) Case H
antihypertensive drugs (an-te-hi-per-ten'siv) Case I
antrum (an'trum) Case H
anulus (an'u-lus) Case F
aorta (a-or'tah) Case I, Plate VIII
aortic (a-or'tik) Case I
aortic insufficiency Case I
apex (a'peks) Case G
apical (ap'e-kal) Case D
appendectomy (ap-en-dek'to-me) Case C
appendiceal (ap-pen-dis-e'al) Case A
appendicitis (ah-pen-di-si'tis) Case A
appendix (ah-pen'diks) Case A, Plate II
areola (ah-re'o-lah); plural, **areolae** (a-re'o-la) Case D
arterial blood gases (ar-te're-al) Case C
arteriolar (ar-te-ri'o-lar) Case G
arteriole (ar-te're-ol) Case G
arteriosclerosis (ar-te-re-o-skle-ro'sis) Case E
arteriosclerotic heart disease (ar-te-re-o-skle-rot'ik) Case G
arthralgia (ar-thral'je-ah) Case D
arthritis (ar-thri'tis) Case D
arthrotomy (ar-throt'o-me) Case I
ascending colon Case H
ascites (ah-si'tez) Case I
asthma (az'mah) Case F
asymptomatic (a-simp-to-mat'ik) Case I
ataxia (a-tak'se-ah) Case I
atelectasis (at-e-lek'tah-sis) Case E
atheroma (ath-er-o'mah) Case I
atheromatous (ath-er-o-'mah-tus) Case I
atrium (a'tre-um) Case I, Plate VIII
atrophy (at'ro-fe) Case G
atypia (a-tip'e-ah) Case G
atypical (a-tip'e-kal) Case I
auditory (aw'de-to-re) Case D
auditory canal (aw'de-to-re) Case E
aural (aw'ral) Case F
auscultation (aws-kul-ta'shun) Case A
autopsy (aw'top-se) Case J
avascular (a-vas'ku-lar) Case D
axilla (ak-sil'ah); plural, **axillae** (ak-sil'a) Case D
axillary (ak'si-lar-e) Case E

B

Babinski (bah-bin'ske) Case A
bacteria (bak-te're-ah) Case E
bacterial (bak-te're-al) Case I
bacteriuria (bak-te-re-u're-ah) Case B
band neutrophil (nu'tro-fil) Case A
barium (ba're-um) Case H
Bartholin's gland (bar'to-linz) Case A
basal (ba'sal) Case C
basement membrane (bas'ment) (mem'bran) Case I
basilar (bas'i-lar) Case E
basilic (ba-sil'ik) Case E
basophil (ba'so-fil) Case A
benign (be-nin') Case B
benign prostatic hypertrophy Case G
bibasilar (bi-bas'i-lar) Case I
bilateral (bi-lat'er-al) Case B
bile (bil) Case A
bile ducts (bil) (dukts) Case J
bilirubin (bil-e-roo'bin) Case H
bimanual (bi-man'u-al) Case D
biopsy (bi'op-se) Case I
bitemporal (bi-tem'po-ral) Case I
bloating (blot'ing) Case J
blood pressure Case A
blood urea nitrogen (blud) (u-re'ah) (ni'tro-jen) Case G
boggy Case B
bowel (bow'el) Case I
broad spectrum Case B
bronchitis (brong-ki'tis) Case F
bronchodilator (brong-ko-di'la-tor) Case G
bronchovascular (brong-ko-vas'ku-lar) Case G
bronchus (brong'kus) Case F, Plate I
bruit (broot'); plural, **bruits** (broots') Case H
buccal (buk'al) Case I
buccal membrane (buk'al) (mem'bran) Case I
bundle branch block Case C

C

calcification (kal-se-fi-ka'shun) Case G
calculus (kal'ku-lus); plural, **calculi** (kal'ku-li) Case A
calyces (ka'li-sez) Case G, Plate IX
cannula (kan'u-lah) Case D
capsule (kap'sul) Case H
carbohydrate (kar-bo-hi'drat) Case H
carbon dioxide (kar'bon) (di-ok'sid) Case D

carcinoma (kar-si-no′mah) Case I
cardiac (kar′de-ak) Case A
cardiac monitor (kar′de-ak) Case G
cardiogram (kar′de-o-gram) Case C
cardiomegaly (kar-de-o-me′ga-le) Case A
cardiorespiratory (kar-de-o-res′pir-ah-to-re) Case A
cardiothoracic (kar-de-o-tho-ras′ic) Case C
cardiothoracic ratio Case C
cardiotonic (kar-de-o-ton′ik) Case I
carotid (kah-rot′id) Case B
cartilage (kar′ti-lij) Case I
cataract (kat′ah-rakt) Case I
catheter (kath′e-ter) Case B
catheterization (kath-e-ter-i-za′shun) Case B
cauda equina (kaw′dah) (e-kwin′ah) Case I
cecum (se′kum) Case A, Plate II
cellular (sel′u-lar) Case G
central venous pressure (ve′nus) Case E
cephalalgia (sef-ah-lal′je-ah) Case I
cervical (ser′ve-kal) Case A
cervical canal Case D
cervix (ser′viks) Case A, Plate X
cesarean section (se-za′re-an) Case H
chemotherapy (ke-mo-ther′ah-pe) Case I
cholecystectomy (ko-le-sis-tek′to-me) Case B
cholelithiasis (ko-le-li-thi′ah-sis) Case G
cholestasis (ko-le-sta′sis) Case J
cholesterol (ko-les′ter-ol) Case G
chorionic (ko-re-on′ik) Case D
chromic catgut (kro′mik) Case A
chronic (kron′ik) Case F
chronically (kron′i-ka-le) Case F
cirrhosis (sir-o′sis) Case J
claudication (klaw-de-ka′shun) Case A
clavicle (klav′e-kl) Case H, Plate III
clonus (klo′nus) Case I
closed reduction Case C
coagulase positive (ko-ag′u-las) Case E
coarctation (ko-ark-ta′shun) Case I
codeine (ko′den) Case C
colic (kol′ik) Case A
colicky (kol′ik-e) Case A
colon (ko′lon) Case C
colonic (ko-lon′ik) Case C
colony count Case B
columnar (ko-lum′nar) Case I

coma (ko′mah) Case B
comatose (ko-mah-tos′) Case B
comminuted (kom′in-ut-ed) Case E
common bile duct (bil) (dukt) Case H
complete blood count Case A
compression (kom-presh′un) Case I
compression fracture (kom-pres′un) (frak′tur) Case I
conception (kon-sep′shun) Case H
conductive hearing loss Case F
congestion (kon-jest′yun) Case F
congestive (kon-jes′tiv) Case G
congestive heart failure (kon-jes′tiv) Case I
consolidation (kon-sol-e-da′shun) Case B
consolidative (kon-sol-e-da′tiv) Case C
consultation (kon-sul-ta′shun) Case H
contraceptives (kon-trah-sep′tivs) Case H
contrast material Case E
contusion (kon-tu′zhun) Case C
convalescence (kon-vah-les′ens) Case A
cornea (kor′ne-ah) Case I, Plate V
coronary (kor′o-na-re) Case J
coronary thrombosis (kor′o-na-re) (throm-bo′sis) Case E
cortex (kor′teks) Case J
cortisone (kor′te-son) Case G
Cortisporin (kor-te-spo′rin) Case F
costal (kos′tal) Case H
costal margin (kos′tal) (mar′jin) Case H
costophrenic (kos-to-fren′ik) Case C
costovertebral angle (kos-to-ver-te′bral) Case A
Coumadin (koo′mah-din) Case C
cranial (kra′ne-al) Case A
cranium (kra′ne-um) Case E
crepitant (krep′i-tant) Case C
crepitant rales (krep′i-tant) (rahls) Case C
crepitus (krep′i-tus) Case E
crest Case E
cross-match Case E
croup (kroop) Case J
croupy (kroop′e) Case J
crypts (kriptz) Case F
cuboidal (ku-boid′al) Case I
culdocentesis (kul-do-sen-te′sis) Case D
culture (kul′tur) Case C
curettage (ku-re-tahzh′) Case D
curette (ku-ret′) Case F
cut down Case E

cutaneous (ku-ta′ne-us) Case C
cyanosis (si-ah-no′sis) Case C
cyanotic (si-ah-not′ik) Case E
cylindrical (sil-in′dre-kl) Case A
cyst (sist) Case I
cystic (sis′tik) Case I
cystitis (sis-ti′tis) Case D
cystogram (sis′to-gram) Case E
cystoscope (sis′to-skop) Case G
cystoscopy (sis-tos′ko-pe) Case G
cystostomy (sis-tos′to-me) Case E
cystotomy (sis-tot′o-me) Case E
cystourethrocele (sis-to-u-re′thro-sel) Case I

D

debilitated (de-bil′li-ta-ted) Case H
debility (de-bil′i-te) Case H
debridement (da-bred-maw′) Case F
decompensation (de-kom-pen-sa′shun) Case D
decompensated (de-kom′pen-sa-ted) Case J
decongestant (de-kon-jes′tant) Case J
deep tendon reflex Case A
degeneration (de-jen-er-a′shun) Case G
degenerative (de-jen′er-a-tiv) Case G
delineate (de-lin′e-at) Case H
demise (de-miz′) Case J
dermatologist (der-mah-tol′o-jist) Case J
dermatology (der-mah-tol′o-je) Case J
descending colon Case H
despondency (de-spon′den-se) Case J
Dexon (dek′son) Case D
diabetes (di-ah-be′tez) Case A
diabetes mellitus (di-ah-be′tez) (mel′i-tus) Case B
diabetic (di-ah-bet′ik) Case B
diaphoresis (di-ah-fo-re′sis) Case I
diaphoretic (di′ah-fo-ret′ik) Case I
diaphragm (di′ah-fram) Case A
diaphragmatic (di-ah-frag-mat′ik) Case C
diarrhea (di-ah-re′ah) Case B
diastolic (di-ah-stol′ik) Case A
differential (dif-er-en′shal) Case C
differentiated (dif-er-en′she-a-ted) Case J
diffuse (de-fus′) Case E
digit (dij′it) Case J
digitalis (dij-e-ta′lis) Case G
digitalized (dij′e-tal-izd) Case G

194

Dilantin (di-lan'ten) Case I
dilation (di-la'shun) Case D
dilate (di'lat) Case D
dilation and curettage Case D
diphtheria (dif-the're-ah) Case J
diplopia (dip-lo'pe-ah) Case I
discharge (dis'charj) Case F
disoriented (dis-o're-en-ted) Case H
dissection (dis-sek'shun) Case D
distal (dis'tal) Case E
distention (dis-ten'shun) Case B
diuretic (di-u-ret'ik) Case I
diverticulitis (di-ver-tik-u-li'tis) Case D
diverticulum (di-ver-tik'u-lum) Case D
dorsal (dor'sal) Case B
dorsal lithotomy position (lith-ot'o-me) Case D
doubly ligated (li'gat-ed) Case E
duodenal (du-o-de'nal) Case G
duodenal loop (du-o-de'nal) (loop) Case H
duodenum (du-o-de'num) Case E, Plate II
dura (du'rah) Case I
dysarthria (dis-ar'thre-ah) Case I
dysfunction (dis-funk'shun) Case J
dysmenorrhea (dis-men-o-re'ah) Case D
dysphagia (dis-fa'je-ah) Case D
dyspnea (disp'ne-ah) Case A
dysuria (dis-u're-ah) Case A

E

ecchymosis (ek-e-mo'sis); plural, **ecchymoses** (ek-e-mo'ses) Case J
ecchymotic (ek-e-mot'ik) Case J
ectopic (ek-top'ik) case D
ectopic gestation (jes-ta'shun) Case D
ectopic pregnancy Case D
eczema (ek'ze-mah) Case J
edema (e-de'mah) Case A
edematous (e-dem'ah-tus) Case F
effusion (ef-u'zhun) Case C
electrocardiogram (e-lek'tro-kar-de-o-gram) Case G
electrocardiographic (e-lek-tro-kar-de-o-gra'fik) Case G
electrocautery (e-lek-tro-kaw'ter-e) Case G
electrolyte (e-lek'tro-lit) Case A
elliptical (e-lip'ti-kal) Case H
emaciated (e-ma'se-a-ted) Case J
embolization (em-bo-li-za'shun) Case C
embolus (em'bo-lus) or **embolism** (em'bo-lizm) Case C
emergency room Case A
emesis (em'e-sis) Case D
emphysema (em-fi-se'mah) Case G
endocarditis (en-do-kar-di'tis) Case I
endocrinology (en-do-krin-ol'o-je) Case B
endotracheal (en-do-tra'ke-al) Case A
engorged (en-gorjd') Case J
engorgement (en-gorj'ment) Case D
enteritis (en-ter-i'tis) Case I
enterocolitis (en-ter-o-ko-li'tis) Case J
enuresis (en-u-re'sis) Case F
enzyme (en'zim) Case J
eosinophil (e-o-sin'o-fil) Case A
epicondylar fracture (ep-e-kon'dil-ar) Case E
epicondyle (ep-e-kon'dil) Case E
epigastric (ep-e-gas'trik) Case C
epiglottis (ep-e-glot'is) Case I, Plates I, VI
epilepsy (ep'e-lep-se) Case I
episiotomy (e-piz-e-ot'o-me) Case H
epistaxis (ep-e-stak'sis) Case I
epithelial (ep-e-the'le-al) Case F
epithelium (ep-e-the'le-um) Case F
erosion (e-ro'zhun) Case I
erythema (er-e-the'mah) Case C
Escherichia coli (esh-er-ik'i-a ko-li) Case B
esophageal (e-sof-ah-je'al) Case J
esophagus (e-sof'ah-gus) Case J, Plate VI
ethanol (eth'ah-nol) Case C
etiology (e-te-ol'o-je) Case I
eustachian tube (u-sta'ke-an) Case F
exacerbation (eg-sas-er-ba'shun) Case H
excise (ek-siz'); past tense, **excised** (ek-sizd) Case A
excision (ek-sizh'un) Case F
excisional (ek-sizh'un-al) Case I
excoriation (eks-ko-re-a'shun) Case I
excretion (eks-kre'shun) Case B
excretory urography (eks'kre-to-re) (u-rog'rah-fe) Case G
excursion (eks-kur'shun) Case C
exogenous (eks-oj'e-nus) Case I
exophthalmos (ek-sof-thal'mus) Case H
exostosis (ek-sos-to'sis) Case I
expiratory wheeze (eks-pir'a-to-re) (hwez) Case G
exquisite (eks'kwi-zit) Case D

external oblique muscle Case A
extradural (eks-trah-du'ral) Case I
extraocular (eks-tra-ok'u-lar) Case C
extrasystole (eks-trah-sis'to-le) Case G
extravasation (eks-trav-ah-sa'shun) Case E
exudate (eks'u-dat) Case A
exudative (eks'u-da-tiv) Case A

F

fallopian tube (fah-lo'pe-an) Case D, Plate X
fascia (fash'e-ah) Case A
febrile (feb'ril) Case B
febrile convulsions (feb'ril) (kon-vul'shunz) Case E
feces (fe'sez) Case G
femoral (fem'or-al) Case B
femur (fe'mur) Case E, Plate IV
fibrocystic disease (fi-bro-sis'tik) Case I
fibromuscular (fi-bro-mus'ku-lar) Case G
fibrosis (fi-bro'sis) Case G
fibrotic (fi-brot'ik) Case J
fifth lumbar vertebra (lum'bar) (ver'te-brah) Case I
figure of eight sutures (su'turz) Case E
fimbria (fim'bre-ah) Case D
fingerbreadths (fing'ger-bredths') Case J
fixation (fiks-a'shun) Case E
fixation pins (fiks-a'shun) Case E
flap Case F
flatplate Case I
flatulence (flat'u-lens) Case B
fleshy Case I
flexion (flek'shun) Case I
fluoroscope (floo-o'ro-skop) Case I
fluoroscopy (floo-or-os'ko-pe) Case I
focal (fo'kal) Case A
Foley catheter (kath'e-ter) Case B
follicles (fol'e-klz) Case J
fossa (fos'ah); plural, **fossae** (fos'a) Case C
fossa ovalis (fos'ah) (o-val'is) Case C
fracture (frak'tur) Case E
friable (fri'ah-bl) Case F
friction rub Case C
frontal lobe (fron'tal) (lob) Case J, Plate VII
fulgurate (ful'gu-rat) Case I
fundus (fun'dus) Case E
funduscopic exam (fun-dus-ko'pik) Case A

G

gait disturbances Case B
gallbladder (gawl′blad-der) Case H, Plate II
gallop Case A
gastric (gas′trik) Case E
gastric vessels (gas′trik) (ves′elz) Case E
gastroenterology (gas-tro-en-ter-ol′o-je) Case H
gastrointestinal (gas-tro-in-tes′tin-al) Case A
Gelfoam (jel′fom) Case F
general anesthesia (an-es-the′ze-ah) Case A
genital (jen′e-tal) Case G
genitalia (jen-e-ta′le-ah) Case I
gestation (jes-ta′shun) Case D
gland (gland) Case G
glandular (glan′du-lar) Case G
glomerulus (glo-mer′u-lus); plural, **glomeruli** (glo-mer′u-li) Case J
gluteal region (gloo′te-al) Case I
glycosuria (gli-ko-su′re-ah) Case B
grade system Case D
gram (gram) Case G
granular (gran′u-lar) Case J
granulation tissue (gran-u-la′shun) (tish′u) Case F
Gravida (grav′id-ah) Case A
greater trochanter (tro-kan′ter) Case J
guaiac (gwi′ak) Case B
gynecologic (gin-e-ko-lo′jik) Case A
gynecologist (gin-e-kol′o-jist) Case D
gynecomastia (jin-e-ko-mas′te-ah) Case J

H

hematemesis (hem-at-em′e-sis) Case A
hematochezia (hem-ah-to-ke′ze-ah) Case D
hematocrit (hem-ah′to-krit) Case A
hematuria (hem-ah-tu′re-ah) Case A
hemoglobin (he-mo-glo′bin) Case A
hemolysis (he-mol′is-is) Case H
hemolytic (he-mo-lit′ik) Case H
hemopneumothorax (he-mo-nu-mo-tho′raks) Case E
hemoptysis (he-mop′tis-is) Case C
hemorrhage (hem′or-ij) Case A
hemorrhagic (hem-o-raj′ik) Case D
hemostasis (he-mos-tah′sis) Case A
hemothorax (he-mo-tho′raks) Case E
Heparin (hep′ah-rin) Case C
hepatic (he-pat′ik) Case J
hepatitis (hep-ah-ti′tis) Case H
hepatomegaly (hep-ah-to-meh′ga-le) Case C
hepatorenal (hep-ah-to-re′nal) Case I
hernia (her′ne-ah) Case F
herniorrhaphy (her-ne-or′ah-fe) Case C
hesitancy (hez′i-ten-se) Case G
hiatal (hi-a′tal) Case J
hiatal hernia (hi-a′tal) (her′ne-ah) Case J
hiatus (hi-a′tus) Case J
histologic (his-to-loj′ik) Case G
histology (his-tol′o-je) Case G
humerus (hu′mer-us) Case E, Plate IV
hydrocephalus (hi-dro-sef′ah-lus) Case F
hydronephrosis (hi-dro-ne-fro′sis) Case G
hyperaeration (hi-per-er-a′shun) Case G
hyperchromatism (hi-per-kro′mah-tizm) Case I
hyperemia (hi-per-e′me-ah) Case G
hyperemesis (hi-per-em′e-sis) Case J
hyperglycemia (hi-per-gli-se′me-ah) Case B
hyperpigmented (hi-per-pig′ment-ed) Case D
hyperplasia (hi-per-pla′ze-ah) Case G
hyperpnea (hi-perp′ne-ah) Case C
hyperpneic (hi-perp′ne-ik) Case B
hyperreflexia (hi-per-re-flek′se-ah) Case J
hyperresonant (hi-per-rez′o-nant) Case G
hypertension (hi-per-ten′shun) Case D
hypertrophic (hi-per-trof′ik) Case F
hypertrophy (hi-per′tro-fe) Case F
hypesthesia (hi-pes-the′ze-ah) Case B
hypoactive (hi-po-ak′tiv) Case B
hypotension (hi-po-ten′shun) Case D
hypotensive (hi-po-ten′siv) Case B
hypotonia (hi-po-to′ne-ah) Case I

I

icteric (ik-ter′ik) Case J
icterus (ik′ter-us) Case B
ileocecal junction (il-e-o-se′kal) Case A
ileum (il′e-um) Case A, Plate II
ileus formation (il′e-us) Case D
ilium (il′e-um) Case E
incision (in-sizh′un) Case E
indirect laryngoscopy (lar-ing-gos′ko-pe) Case I
induration (in-du-ra′shun) Case C
infarct (in′farkt) **infarction** (in-fark′shun) Case C
infectious (in-fek′shus) Case H
infiltrate (in-fil′trat) Case C
infiltrated (in-fil′trat-ed) Case F
infiltration (in-fil-tra′shun) Case A
inflammatory cells (in-flam′ah-to-re) Case G
ingestion (in-jes′chun) Case B
inguinal (ing′gwi-nal) Case C
injected (in-jekt′ed) Case A
insufflated (in′suf-fla-ted) Case D
insulin (in′su-lin) Case B
intensive care unit Case C
intercostal (in-ter-kos′tal) Case B
intermittent positive pressure breathing Case E
internal oblique muscle Case A
interspace (in′ter-spas) Case I
interstitial (in-ter-stish′al) Case G
intestine (in-tes′tin) Case A, Plate II
intracranial (in-trah-kra′ne-al) Case I
intramuscularly (in-trah-mus′ku-lar-le) Case I
intraperitoneal (in-trah-per-e-to-ne′al) Case D
intravenous (in-trah-ve′nus) Case B
intravenous pyelogram (in-trah-ve′nus) (pi′el-o-gram) Case B
intubate (in′tu-bat) Case F
invasion (in-va′zhun) Case I
iris (i′ris); plural, **irides** (i′rid-ez) Case J, Plate V
irrigated (ir′i-gat-ed) Case G
ischemia (is-ke′me-ah) Case C
isophane insulin suspension Case B
isotope (i′so-top) Case C
isthmus (isth′mus) Case D

J

jaundice (jawn′dis) Case A
jaundiced (jawn′dist) Case J
jugular (jug′u-lar) Case C
jugular venous pulse Case I

K

Keflex (ke′fleks) Case B
Kelly clamp Case A
keratin (ker′ah-tin) Case F
ketoacidosis (ke-to-as-e-do′sis) Case B

L

labile (la′bil) Case J
labium majora (la′be-um) (mah-jo′rah) Case I
lacerated (las′er-at-ed) Case E
laceration (las-er-a′shun) Case E
laminar (lam′i-nar) Case G
laparoscope (lap′ah-ro-skop) Case D
laparoscopy (lap-ah-ros′ko-pe) Case D
laparotomy (lap-ah-rot′o-me) Case D
laryngoscopy (lar-ing-gos′ko-pe) Case I
larynx (lar′inks) Case I, Plates I, VI
lateral (lat′er-al) Case C
lavage (lah-vahzh′) Case E
LDH Case H
lesion (le′zhun) Case A
lesser sac (sak) Case E
leukocyte (lu′ko-sit) Case A
leukocytosis (lu-ko-si-to′sis) Case A
leukopenia (lu-ko-pen′e-ah) Case H
leukoplakia (lu-ko-pla′ke-ah) Case I
ligament (lig′ah-ment) Case D
ligate (li′gat) Case A
ligatures (lig′a-churs) Case A
liter (le′ter) Case D
lithotomy (lith-ot′o-me) Case D
livor mortis (li′vor) (mor′tis) Case J
lobe (lob) Case G
lordosis (lor-do′sis) Case I
lucent (lu′sent) Case J
lumbar (lum′bar) Case D
lumbar vertebra, 3rd, 4th, 5th, Case I
lumen (lu′men) Case D
lymph (limf) Case D
lymphadenopathy (lim-fad-e-nop′ah-the) Case D
lymph gland Case D
lymphocyte (lim′fo-sit) Case A
lymphoid (lim′foid) Case F
lysis (li′sis) Case H

M

macula (mak′u-lah) Case B
maculopapular (mak-u-lo-pap′u-lar) Case I
malignancy (mah-lig′nan-se) Case F
malleolus (mal-e′o-lus) Case B
mammography (mam-og′rah-fe) Case I
mass (mas) Case C
mastoid (mas′toid) Case F, Plate VII
mastoidectomy (mas-toid-ek′to-me) Case F
McBurney incision Case A
meatal (me-a′tal) Case J
meatus (me-a′tus) Case D
medial (me′de-al) Case J
mediastinum (me-de-as-ti′num) Case J
medulla (me-dul′ah) Case E
medullary (med′u-lar-e) Case E
melena (mel′e-na) Case B
membrane (mem′bran) Case A
menorrhagia (men-or-ra′je-ah) Case D
mesenteric (mes-en-ter′ik) Case A
mesoappendix (mes-o-ah-pen′diks) Case A
mesosalpinx (mes-o-sal′pinks) Case D
metabolic (met-ah-bol′ik) Case G
metabolism (me-tab′o-lizm) Case G
metastasis (me-tas′tah-sis); plural, **metastases** (me-tas′tah-ses) Case I
metastatic (met-ah-stat′ik) Case I
metrorrhagia (met-ro-ra′je-ah) Case D
microgram (mi′kro-gram) Case J
microscopic (mi-kro-skop′ik) Case J
midclavicular (mid-klah-vik′u-lar) Case B
midline Case A
midshaft Case E
migraine (mi′gran) Case I
millimeter (mil′e-me-ter) Case D
mitosis (mi-to′sis) Case J
mitral (mi′tral) Case D
mitral insufficiency Case D
monitoring (mon′i-tor-ing) Case E
motility (mo-til′i-te) Case H
mouth gag Case F
mucin (mu′sin) Case I
mucosa (mu-ko′sah) Case D
murmur (mur′mur) Case A
muscle guarding Case A
myelogram (mi′el-o-gram) Case I
myocardial (mi-o-kar′de-al) Case C
myocardium (mi-o-kar′de-um) Case C
myxedema (mik-se-de′mah) Case I

N

naris (na′ris); plural, **nares** (na′res) Case E
nasopharynx (na-zo-far′inks) Case F
necrosis (ne-kro′sis) Case I
neoplasia (ne-o-pla′ze-ah) Case G
nephritis (ne-fri′tis) Case I
nephropathy (nef-rop′ah-the) Case I
nephrotoxic (nef-ro-tok′sik) Case I
neuritis (nu-ri′tis) Case J
neurological (nu-ro-loj′e-kal) Case I
neutrophil (nu′tro-fil) Case A
nevus (ne′vus) Case I
nitroglycerine (ni-tro-glis′er-in) Case G
nocturia (nok-tu′re-ah) Case A
nodes (nodz) Case D
nodular (nod′u-lar) Case J
nodule (nod′ul) Case J
noncontributory Case E
normal saline (sa′len) Case D
normocephalic (nor-mo-se-fal′ik) Case A
NPH Case B
nucleus (nu′kle-us); plural, **nuclei** (nu′kle-i) Case I

O

obese (o-bes′) Case I
obesity (o-bes′i-te) Case I
obstipation (ob-sti-pa′shun) Case I
obtunded (ob-tund′ed) Case B
occiput (ok′si-put) Case J
occluded (ok-klud′ed) Case G
ocular (ok′u-lar) Case B
opacify (o-pas′i-fi); past tense, **opacified** (o-pas′i-fid) Case H
ophthalmoscopic (of-thal-mo-skop′ik) Case D
oral contraceptive (kon-trah-sep′tiv) Case D
orally (o′ral-le) Case A
organism (or′gan-ism) Case E
organomegaly (or-gan-o-me′ga-le) Case A
orifice (or′i-fis); plural, **orifices** (or′i-fi-sez) Case G
oropharynx (o-ro-far′inks) Case C
orthopedic (or-tho-pe′dik) Case E
orthopedic surgeon (or-tho-pe′dik) Case E
orthopnea (or-thop′ne-ah) Case B
osteomyelitis (os-te-o-mi-e-li′tis) Case E
ostium (os′te-um); plural, **ostia** (os′te-ah) Case J
outpatient (out′pa-shent) Case D
ovary (o′vah-re) Case D, Plate X

P

palate (pal′at) Case F
palpable (pal′pah-bl) Case D
palpated (pal′pat-ed) Case E
palpitations (pal-pi-ta′shunz) Case D
pancreas (pan′kre-as) Case I, Plate II

197

panendoscope (pan-en'do-skop) Case G
papillary (pap'i-ler-e) Case I
papilledema (pap-i-le-de'mah) Case I
Para (pa'ra) Case A
paralysis (pah-ral'is-is) Case I
parametrial (par-ah-me'tre-al) Case I
parametrium (par-ah-me'tre-um) Case I
paravertebral (par-ah-ver'te-bral) Case H
parenteral (par-en'ter-al) Case H
paresis (pah-re'sis) or (par'e-sis) Case I
paresthesias (par-es-the'ze-as) Case B
paroxysmal (par-ok-siz'mal) Case J
partial pressure of carbon dioxide Case C
partial pressure of oxygen Case C
patent (pa'tent) Case J
pathogen (path'o-jen) Case C
pathological (path-o-loj'e-kal) Case D
pathology (pah-thol'o-je) Case D
pCO2 Case C
pedal (ped'al) Case B
pedicle (ped'e-kel) Case E
pedunculated (pe-dung'ku-lat-ed) Case I
pelvic (pel'vik) Case D
pelvis (pel'vis) Case D
penicillin (pen-e-sil'in) Case C
Penrose drain Case E
percussion (per-kush'un) Case A
perforation (per-fo-ra'shun) Case E
perfusion (per-fu'zhun) Case C
per high-powered field Case J
pericardial (per-e-kar'de-al) Case I
periosteal (per-e-os'te-al) Case J
periosteum (per-e-os'te-um) Case J
peripheral (peh-rif'er-al) Case E
peripheral neuritis (peh-rif'er-al) (nu-ri'tis) Case J
peritoneal (per-i-to-ne'al) Case A
peritoneal cavity Case D
peritoneum (per-i-to-ne'um) Case A
peritonitis (per-i-to-ni'tis) Case D
pertussis (per-tus'is) Case J
pes planus (pez) (pla'nus) Case F
petechiae (pe-te'ke-i) Case F
Pfannenstiel incision (pfahn'en-stel) Case D
phallus (fal'us) Case B
phenobarbital (fe-no-bar'bi-tal) Case I
phenol (fe'nol) Case A
philtrum (fil'trum) Case E
phlebitis (fle-bi'tis) Case H

phlebolith (fleb'o-lith) Case G
pigmented (pig-ment'ed) Case I
pitting edema (e-de'mah) Case J
placenta (plah-sen'tah) Case H
placenta previa (plah-sen'tah) (pre've-ah) Case H
plasma cells (plaz'mah) Case F
pleomorphism (ple-o-mor'fism) Case J
pleura (ploor'ah) Case C
pleural (ploor'al) Case C
pleurisy (ploor'i-se) Case C
pleuritic (ploor-it'ik) Case C
pneumonia (nu-mo'ne-ah) Case I
pneumonic (nu-mon'ik) Case C
pneumonitis (nu-mo-ni'tis) Case C
pneumothorax (nu-mo-tho'raks) Case E
pO2 Case C
point of maximum impulse Case B
poly (pol'e) Case F
polydipsia (pol-e-dip'se-ah) Case C
polyp (pol'ip) Case C
polyphagia (pol-e-fa'je-ah) Case C
polypoid (pol'e-poid) Case F
polyuria (pol-e-u're-ah) Case C
popliteal (pop-lit-e'al) Case B
porta hepatis (por'tah) (he-pat'is) Case E
portable Case E
posterior (pos-te're-or) Case C
posteroanterior (pos'ter-o-an-ter'e-or) Case C
postoperative Case A
postpartum (post-par'tum) Case H
prepped Case A
prescription (pre-skrip'shun) Case H
presumptive diagnosis (pre-zump'tiv) (di-ag-no'sis) Case G
prior to admission Case A
proctoscopy (prok-tos'ko-pe) Case H
productive cough (pro-duk'tiv) (kawf) Case G
prognosis (prog-no'sis) Case G
projections (pro-jek'shuns) Case I
promontory (prom'on-to-re) Case F
prophylactic (pro-fi-lak'tik) Case D
proprioception (pro-pre-o-sep'shun) Case J
prostate (pros'tat) Case B
prostatic (pros-tat'ik) Case G
prostatitis (pros-tah-ti'tis) Case B
prosthesis (pros-the'sis) Case J
prosthetic (pros-thet'ik) Case J
protein (pro'te-in) Case H
proteus (pro'te-us) Case E
prothrombin (pro-throm'bin) Case C
prothrombin time Case C
protuberant (pro-tu'ber-ant) Case J

pruritus (proo-ri'tis) Case I
psoas (so'as) Case B
psychiatrist (si-ki'ah-trist) Case J
ptosis (to'sis) Case I
pubic bone (pu'bik) Case A
pubis (pu'bis) Case E
pulmonary (pul'mo-na-re) Case A
pulmonic (pul-mon'ik) Case C
punch forcep (punch) (for'sep) Case F
punctate (punk'tat) Case B
pupil (pu'pil) Case G, Plate V
purulent (pu'roo-lent) Case F
pyelocalyceal (pi-el-o-kal-e-se'al) Case B
pyelogram (pi'el-o-gram) Case G
pyelonephritis (pi-el-o-ne-fri'tis) Case I
pylorus (pi-lo'rus) Case H
pyuria (pi-u're-ah) Case B

Q

quadrant (kwod'rant) Case A

R

radiation of pain Case A
radiation therapy (ra-de-a'shun) (ther'ah-pe) Case I
rales (rahls) Case B
rebound tenderness Case A
recrudescence (re-kroo-des'ens) Case I
rectally (rek'tal-le) Case B
rectus fascia (rek'tus) (fash'e-ah) Case E
rectus muscles (rek'tus) Case D
red blood cells Case J
reflex (re'fleks); plural, **reflexes** (re'fleks-is) Case D
reflux (re'fluks) Case H
regimen (rej'i-men) Case H
regurgitation (re-gur-ji-ta'shun) Case I
renal (re'nal) Case A
reprepped and redraped Case D
resect (re-sekt') Case D
resection (re-sek'shun) Case G
resectoscope (re-sek'to-skop) Case G
respiration (res-pi-ra'shun) Case A
respiratory (re-spir'ah-to-re) Case A
resuscitate (re-sus'i-tat) Case J
resuscitative (re-sus-i-ta'tiv) Case J
retardation (re-tar-da'shun) Case F
retention sutures Case E
retina (ret'i-nah) Case I, Plate V

retinal (ret′i-nel) Case B
retinopathy (ret-i-nop′ah-the) Case B
retracting (re-trak′ting) Case D
retroperitoneal (re-tro-per-i-to-ne′al) Case E
rheumatic (ru-mat′ik) Case D
rheumatic heart disease Case D
rheumatism (ru′mah-tizm) Case D
rheumatoid (ru′mah-toid) Case D
rhinitis (ri-ni′tis) Case A
Romberg (rom′berg) Case C
Romberg test Case J
rhonchi (rong′ki) Case B
right bundle branch block Case C
rigor mortis (ri′gor) (mor′tis) Case J
Ringer's lactate (lak′tat) Case B
Rinne test (ren-e′) Case J
roentgen (rent′gen) Case J
roseola (ro-ze-o′lah) Case F
round ligament Case D
rubella (roo-bel′ah) Case A
rule out Case C
rupture (rup′chur) Case D

S

sacroiliac joint (sa-kro-il′e-ak) Case E
sacrum (sa′krum) Case E
saline (sa′len) Case D
salpingectomy (sal-pin-jek′to-me) Case D
sanguineous (sang-gwin′e-us) Case H
scan Case C
scapula (skap′u-lah) Case I
Scarlet fever Case A
sclerae (skle′ra) Case A, Plate V
scleral (skle′ral) Case H
scoliosis (sko-le-o′sis) Case D
scout film Case H
seborrhea (seb-o-re′ah) Case J
sedation (se-da′shun) Case I
sediment (sed′i-ment) Case J
sedimentation rate (sed-i-men-ta′shun) Case F
segmented neutrophil (nu′tro-fil) Case A
seizure (se′zhur) Case J
semicomatose (sem-e-ko-mah-tos′) Case E
sensitivity (sen-si-tiv′i-te) Case E
sensorium (sen-so′re-um) Case J
sequelae (se-kwe′li) Case B
serosa (se-ro′sah) Case A
serosal (se-ro′sal) Case A
serosanguineous (se-ro-sang-gwin′-e-us) Case H

serous (se′rus) Case H
serum (se′rum) Case A
serum electrolytes (e-lek′tro-litz) Case A
SGOT Case H
SGPT Case H
shifting dullness Case J
shock (shok) Case E
shock trauma unit Case E
shocky (sho′ke) Case D
sibling (sib′ling) Case D
sigmoid (sig′moid) Case C
sigmoidoscope (sig-moid-o-skop′) Case C
sigmoidoscopic (sig-moid-os-kop′ik) Case C
sigmoidoscopy (sig-moid-os′ko-pe) Case H
sinus (si′nus) Case B
sinus rhythm (si′nus) Case A
sinus tachycardia (tak-e-kar′de-ah) Case B
Skene's gland (skenz) Case A
snare loop Case I
soft palate (pal′at) Case F
sphincter (sfingk′ter) Case B
spinal anesthetic (spi′nal) (an-es-thet′ik) Case G
spleen (splen) Case E, Plate II
splenectomy (sple-nek′to-me) Case E
splenic (splen′ik) Case E
splenomegaly (sple-no-meg′ah-le) Case G
spotty (spot′e) Case D
sputum (spu′tum) Case C
squamous (skwa′mus) Case F
stab incision Case E
stabilizing pins Case E
stalk (stawk) Case I
staphylococcus aureus (staf-i-lo-kok′kus) (aw′re-us) Case E
stenosis (ste-no′sis) Case J
sterile saline (ster′il) (sa′len) Case E
sternum (ster′num) Case I, Plate III
stool (stool) Case I
strabismus (strah-biz′mus) Case I
stroma (stro′mah) Case F
subacute (sub-ah-kut′) Case I
subcostal (sub-kos′tal) Case H
subcutaneous (sub-ku-ta′ne-us) Case A
subcuticular (sub-ku-tik′u-lar) Case D
sublingual (sub-ling′gual) Case G
substernal (sub-ster′nal) Case I
subumbilical (sub-um-bil′e-kal) Case D

sulcus (sul′kus); plural, **sulci** (sul′si) Case C
sulfa drugs (sul′fah) Case I
supine (su-pin′) Case A
suppurative (sup′u-ra-tiv) Case A
supraclavicular (su-prah-klah-vik′u-lar) Case H
suprapubic (su-prah-pu′bik) Case E
suture (su′tur) Case A
symmetrical (si-met′re-kal) Case F
sympathectomy (sim-pah-thek′to-me) Case I
sympathetic nerves (sim-pah-thet′ik) (nervz) Case I
symphysis (sim′fi-sis) Case E
symphysis pubis (sim′fi-sis) (pu′bis) Case E
symptoms (simp′tums) Case D
syncope (sin′ko-pe) Case J
syndrome (sin′drom) Case I
systolic (sis-tol′ik) Case A

T

tachycardia (tak-e-kar′de-ah) Case B
tachypnea (tak-ip′ne-ah) Case H
temporal (tem′po-ral) Case, I, Plate VII
tenaculum (te-nak′u-lum) Case D
tendon (ten′dun) Case B
testes (tes′tes) Case B
testicular (tes-tik′u-lar) Case G
thoracic (tho-ras′ik) Case E
thoracic vertebra, 11th, Case I
thorax (tho′raks) Case A
thrill Case A
thrombophlebitis (throm-bo-fle-bi′tis) Case C
thrombosis (throm-bo′sis) Case E
thyroid (thi′roid) Case C
tibia (tib′e-ah) Case C, Plate IV
tinnitus (tin′i-tus) Case I
tissue (tish′u) Case A
tonsillectomy (ton-si-lek′to-me) Case A
tonsillitis (ton-si-li′tis) Case D
tonsils (ton′silz) Case D
torus tubarius (to′rus) (tu-ba′re-us) Case F
trabeculae (trah-bek′u-la) Case G
trachea (tra′ke-ah) Case A, Plates I, VI
tracheostomy (tra-ke-os′to-me) Case E
traction (trak′shun) Case E
transcanal (trans-ka-nal′) Case F
transfusion (trans-fu′zhun) Case E
transfusions (trans-fu′zhunz) Case H

transient (tran′shent) Case I
transurethral (trans-u-re′thral) Case G
transversalis fascia (trans-ver-sa′lis) (fash′yah) Case A
transverse (trans-vers′) Case E
transverse colon Case H
transversus muscle (trans-ver′sus) Case A
trapezius muscles (trah-pe′ze-us) Case J
trauma (traw′mah) Case B
tricuspid (tri-kus′pid) Case J
trigone (tri′gon) Case G
trilobar (tri-lo′bar) Case G
trochanter (tro-kan′ter) Case J
trophic (trof′ik) Case B
tubal (tu′bal) Case D
tubal pregnancy Case D
tubal stump Case D
tuberculosis (tu-ber-ku-lo′sis) Case A
tubules (tu′bulz) Case J
tumor (tu′mor) Case J
turbinate (tur′bi-nat) Case J
turgor (tur′gor) Case I
two plus enlarged Case C
Tylenol (ti′le-nol) Case F
tympanic membranes (tim-pan′ik) Case E
tympano-mastoiditis (tim-pah-no-mas-toid-i′tis) Case F
tympanotomy (tim-pah-not′o-me) Case F

typed Case E

U

ulcer (ul′ser) Case G
umbilicus (um-bi-li′kus) Case A
upper gastointestinal series Case G
upright (up′rit) Case D
ureter (u′re-ter) Case B, Plate IX
ureteral (u-re′ter-al) Case A
ureterovesical junction (u-re-ter-o-ves′e-kal) Case G
urethra (u-re′thrah) Case A, Plate IX
urethral (u-re′thral) Case D
urethral sounds (u-re′thral) Case G
urinary (u′ri-ner-e) Case A
urinary retention (u′ri-ner-e) (re-ten′shun) Case G
urology (u-rol′o-je) Case E
uterine (u′ter-in) Case D
uterus (u′ter-us) Case A, Plate X
uvula (u′vu-lah) Case F

V

vaginal (vaj′i-nal) Case D, Plate X
varicella (var-i-sel′ah) Case A
varices (var′i-sez) Case J
varicocele (var′e-ko-sel) Case C
varicose (var-e-kos′) Case C
varicosities (var-e-kos′i-tez) Case C
vascularity (vas-ku-lar′i-te) Case A

vascularized (vas′ku-la-rizd) Case F
vasculature (vas′ku-la-tur) Case A
venous (ve′nus) Case B
ventricle (ven′tre-kl) Case C, Plate VIII
ventricular (ven-trik′u-lar) Case C
vertebra (ver′te-brah); plural, **vertebrae** (ver′te-bra) Case I, Plate III
vertigo (ver′te-go) Case B
verumontanum (ver-ru-mon-ta′num) Case G
vesicle (ves′e-kal) Case G
vesicle outlet obstruction Case G
villi (vil′e) Case D
viral (vi′ral) Case E
visceromegaly (vis-er-o-meg′a-le) Case J
visual (vizh′u-al) Case D
vital signs Case C
void Case B
vulva (vul′vah) Case I

W

wheeze (hwez) Case I
white blood cell Case A
white blood count Case B
white matter Case J
within normal limits Case A

X

xiphoid (zif′oid) Case E
Xylocaine (zi′lo-kan) Case F

0-538-11490-8